W9-AOL-985

INFECTION
prevention and control

INFECTION
prevention and control

ELAINE C. DUBAY, R.N., B.S.

Nurse Epidemiologist, Infection Control Department,
Tucson Medical Center, Tucson, Arizona

REBA D. GRUBB

Medical Writer, Tucson Medical Center, Tucson, Arizona

with 40 illustrations

THE C. V. MOSBY COMPANY

SAINT LOUIS   1973

Printed in the United States of America

Distributed in Great Britain by Henry Kimpton, London

Library of Congress Cataloging in Publication Data

Dubay, Elaine C
   Infection: prevention and control.

    1. Hospitals—Hygiene. 2. Cross infection.
I. Grubb, Reba D., 1916-   joint author.
II. Title [DNLM: 1. Communicable disease control.
2. Cross infection—Prevention and control. WX 165
D813i 1973]
RA969.D8   614.4'4   73-1442
ISBN 0-8016-1466-X

VH/M/M 9 8 7 6 5 4 3 2

To all who have helped through knowledge or patient care
to improve the practice of infection prevention and control
in hospitals and related institutions.

Elaine C. Dubay

To Pauline Zelickson, Rachel Pepperd, Edith Fawver,
Henrietta Corley, Marlyn Pride, and Margaret Blattman,
my deepest gratitude for their constant encouragement and friendship.

Reba D. Grubb

Foreword

Renewed awareness of the toll already being imposed by nosocomial infections flickered into being nearly two decades ago. Gratuitous evidence accumulated slowly but became overwhelming and finally prompted investigation which illuminated the obscurity that had prevailed. The implications of these disclosures aroused interest that evolved into concern. As the problem took on sharper definition, its genesis was explained and its magnitude was explored and described. The need for active, comprehensive programs for control and prevention in every health care facility was validated and acknowledged to be imperative.

Initial approaches were tentative, sporadic. Improvements followed; infection control committees were formed. Later, during the middle and late 1960's, circumstances prompted creation of a new professional health category in which the principal staff members are the infection control nurse and the hospital epidemiologist. They worked hard, but they worked in a situation that still was not fully understood. Success, although becoming attainable, was elusive. Since then the number of persons engaged in this work has grown and continues to grow steadily. Success has become more frequent, but it is still elusive.

In 1969 the Center for Disease Control in Atlanta, Georgia, began a continuing program of surveillance of nosocomial infections in selected hospitals across the nation. Contemporary follow-up indicates that at least 10 percent of all patients admitted to hospitals for short-term periods have clinical infections of one kind or another when they enter. This 10 percent constitutes one reservoir of infection. From this and other reservoirs, an additional 5 percent *acquire* infections during their stay. It is the causes of this acquisition that are of immediate concern.

Obviously, there is room for radical improvement in many instances; the overall rate can certainly be reduced—but only by reducing the inadmissible rates still to be found in certain individual institutions. This reduction *can* be effected. Certain infection control programs are known to have had admirable results. Those of other institutions leave something to be desired despite sincere efforts. Some institutions still have no program at all; others only pay lip service to paper programs.

However, even when high transmission rates are patently the result of inadequately executed control measures or of mere lip service to such measures, scrutiny of the circumstances frequently discloses a still more fundamental cause—lack of knowledge, which may masquerade as disinterest, lethargy, or even irresponsibility. Whatever the mask presented, the basic shortcoming lies in the lack of knowledge of the seriousness of the risks being incurred and, more important, in the lack of the specialized information that can make reduction of these risks feasible. Such information can make it possible to recognize or develop reliable procedures, to adapt uniform procedures to local situations, to establish and maintain practicable programs, to select those persons who can adequately discharge responsibility, and to administer a program effectively.

This volume is intended to fill many gaps in this specialized knowledge. The authors have drawn on both experience and research findings to suggest a basis for workable, effective control of infections. Their ideas and methods are applicable in any institution, large or small, whether it provides general or special care, for short periods or long. The information given here is intended primarily for that new category of health worker exemplified by the infection control nurse and the hospital epidemiologist, but it is no less important to all professional workers in health care facilities.

Used as a reference, this book will prove to be a valuable aid for persons already trained and experienced in infection control work; used as a text, it can provide essential background information for persons whose work is less specialized and for those who are newcomers to the health care field.

Rudolf G. Wanner, M.D., M.P.H.
Medical Training Officer,
Training Program, Center for Disease Control,
Atlanta, Georgia

Preface

Many diseases probably existed millions of years before man inhabited the earth. With the progress of civilization, *man's* contact with *man* has been the prime factor in the spread of disease. From his earliest days he has tried a variety of methods, often cruel and not always successful, to prevent, cure, and control disease. As man has learned to cure a particular disease or to correct one problem by surgery, he has sometimes unintentionally created another. It was true that all too often the operation was a success but the patient died of a secondary infection. Man's greatest steps forward in battling infection have come with the administration of direct patient care and control of the patient's environment.

The sign of Apollo, which citizens of ancient Greece placed on their doors, gave little protection against the diseases that came from the filth in which they lived and the contaminated water that they drank. Protection became a reality only when they cleaned up their environment and their water supply.

Today, the processes of pasteurization, sterilization, and purification do their share to prevent and control infection. The daily routine measures of prevention and control taken by the general public are generally effective when consistently used; but they are not enough in hospitals and other health facilities. Infection is a problem in this environment as it is nowhere else. The ill, the newborn, and the geriatric are more susceptible to infection because they have less resistance. The same germs that may be harmless or of minor consequence to a well-functioning person may cause serious setbacks and even death in the patient with low resistance. In the mid-1800's the risk of postoperative infection in the hospital was so great that Sir James Simpson, the discoverer of chloroform, observed that the man lying on the operating table in one of the surgical hospitals was exposed to a greater risk of death than was the English soldier on the field at Waterloo. Dr. Charles Bell, a distinguished nineteenth century Edinburgh surgeon, went so far as to call the hospital "the house of death." He believed that a physician gave his patients a better chance of recovery by hurrying them out of the hospital to a fresher, cleaner environment.

Health facilities will probably never be completely free of infection because they exist to administer to the ill. Disease and infection are ever present, and for this reason every effort must be made to keep the institutional environment as germ-free as possible. In no other way can the patients who must temporarily live in this environment or the staff administering to their needs be protected from the spread of infection.

Prevention and control of the spread of infection demand a relentless battle and constant attention. Primitive man was not far amiss in his belief that illness was caused by the entrance of evil spirits or devils into a person's body, since disease germs can be "devils" in their actions. They are prepared to take advantage of every opportunity to perform their deadly work.

In this text, the discussion of the battle against infection in the institutional environment is divided into two areas: prevention and control. There is, as there should be, some overlapping of these areas. The division is somewhat arbitrarily made in an effort to point out and deal with the problem of infection in every facet of the organization.

Prevention as defined in this book has two goals: first, it aims at protecting the uninfected patient from any disease or infection; second, it tries to forestall in the patient any increase in preexisting infection of a noncommunicable nature.

Control as defined in this book has the following goals: to check the spread of a preexisting communicable or infectious disease to other patients, visitors, or personnel; to limit the disease so that it does not become more serious in the patient already infected with a communicable disease; and to keep the highly susceptible patient with no present disease from becoming infected.

The goal of prevention and control is reached through specific and general policies and procedures. A *policy* is practical wisdom—any governing principle, plan, or course of action. A *procedure* is the action taken or the manner of accomplishing this course of action; it is the step, or steps, taken to proceed. The elements of policies and procedures are interrelated and must work together.

Policies and procedures for prevention and control of disease and infection are not an innovation. Early examples, although strange to us, were apparently logical to those who determined and used them. Although sometimes extreme and ineffective, they were at least efforts at prevention and control and showed that the need for such measures existed.

During the plague of the early eighteenth century, the policy of prevention was to remove the patient, who was considered to be the source of infection, to a field where he would either recover or die. Those who cared for the patient were then isolated for ten days after the patient either died or recovered.

The people of that time believed that the foul air caused spread of the plague. Physicians courageous enough to care for the sick protected themselves as best they could with gowns, masks, and gloves. They were attired in helmets, long robes, and heavy gauntlets. Their faces were protected with large glasses and a respirator, resembling a long beak filled with aromatic herbs.

The aftermath of the San Francisco earthquake in 1906 was a chaos of death, injury, disease, and destruction. The fear of a typhoid epidemic was very real with the dead and dying lining the streets. Food, water, and shelter were scarce, and most available supplies were contaminated. Strict ordinances (or policies) were enforced by the military. The procedure was extreme and unbending; anyone disobeying the rules was shot.

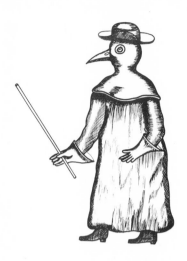

Protective garb dating from 1721. Redrawn from a plate of the frontispiece from *Relation de la peste de Marseilles, Plague of Marseilles,* 1721.

Today, health facilities, regardless of the size and structure, are less extreme in their approach to enforcing policies of prevention and control. Instead of fear and punishment they have established a good, strong system of knowledge through education. These programs of infection control and prevention are further reinforced through written up-to-date policies and procedures that are made available to every staff member of the health care facility.

This we believe is our power structure to keep the threat of disease at a minimum. Strict adherence to these policies and procedures is a must for all personnel, medical staff, students, and visitors. Only when we have full cooperation can the prevention and control of infection be achieved.

We are indebted to many friends and colleagues who have advised either directly or indirectly about the content of the book. They include Dr. R. E. Hastings (surgeon and past chairman of the Infection Control Committee, Tucson Medical Center); Dr. Stewart Westfall (internist); Dr. Charles Pullen (pediatrician); Dr. George Fraser (gynecologist); Dr. George King (general practitioner); Dr. Clifford Hoffman (urologist); Elizabeth Phillips, R.N. (personnel health); Ruth Combecker, R.N. (Supervisor, Visiting Nurse Association, Tucson Division); Dr. Ronald Almgren (the first chairman of Tucson's Inter-Hospital Infection Control Committee); Walter Cheifetz (attorney, firm of Lewis and Roca, Phoenix, Arizona); Sister

Kathleen Clark, CSC (nurse epidemiologist, St. Joseph's Hospital, Tucson); George Mallison (Chief, Microbiologic Section, Center for Disease Control, Atlanta, Georgia).

Our special gratitude goes to Tucson Medical Center and its staff, especially Donald G. Shropshire (Administrator); Marie Booth, R.N. (Administrator, Patient Care Division); Beatrice Mason, R.N. (Director of Nursing Service); Lilah Harper, R.N. (Director, Nursing Research and Products); Jane Mueller, R.N. (Coordinator of Education); Dr. Robert Armstrong (pathologist); Patricia Synder, R.N. (Director, Obstetrics Nursing); Fred Mueller (Director, Environmental Services); Margit Hanson, R.N. (Supervisor, Central Service); Geraldine Ondor, R.N. (Operating Room Education Coordinator); Enola Palmer, R.N., and Anneliese Dickhoff, R.N. (I.V. nurses); Richard Kinney, R.P.H. (pharmacist); Orpha Berrie, R.N. (Head Nurse, Isolation Wing); Larry Inman (traction technician); Barbara Springate (dietitian); Steve McPherson (Director, Respiratory Therapy); Linda Alpert, R.N. (Director, Chest Clinic); Tom Burk and George Ball (medical photography); Jerry Freund (Director of Education); Tom Krug (Assistant Director of Education); and Ruby Gerg (isolation technician).

For their valuable assistance in research, we wish to thank Helen Turner and Kelly Hastings, medical librarians, Tucson Medical Center, and Anita Tschida, librarian, College of Medicine Library, University of Arizona. For their editorial assistance we thank Jean Kingsley and Pamela Mayhall, who was also the major contributor to Chapter 3.

A very special thank you to Dr. Rudolf Wanner, Medical Training Officer, Training Program, Center for Disease Control, for his help and encouragement; to Dr. Mary Fried, Chief Microbiologist, Tucson Medical Center, who was a major contributor to Chapter 1, for sharing her knowledge of germs with us; to artist Travis L. Mayhall for his excellent illustrations; and to Tony Mazel, Pima County Public Health Environmentalist.

Elaine C. Dubay
Reba D. Grubb

Contents

1 Microorganisms and infection, 1

Bacteria, 1
  Optimum conditions, 1
  Morphology, 3
  Reproduction, 4
  Sporulation, 4
  Staining, 4
Normal flora, 5
  Mouth, 7
  Throat, 7
  Nasopharynx, 7
  Trachea, bronchi, lungs, and accessory nasal and mastoid sinuses, 7
  Stomach, 7
  Duodenum, 8
  Below the duodenum, 8
  Genitourinary tract, 9
  Skin, 9
  Other areas, 9
Pathogens, 9
Epidemiology of infection, 10
Body's natural defenses, 14
Community- and hospital-associated infections, 16
  Classification of infections, 17

2 Infection control structure and organization, 19

Infection control committee, 19
  Committee membership, 21
  Functions, 21
Role of the nurse epidemiologist, 22
  Qualifications, 23
  Functions, 24

3 Developing the surveillance program, 25

Role of the nurse and physician, 25
Personnel health service program, 26
  Preemployment examination, 26
  Immunizations, 26
  Follow-up, 26

Other services, 27
Health service nurse, 27
Records, 28
Policies and procedures for prevention and control, 28
Prevention policies and procedures, 29
Control (isolation) policies and procedures, 45
Categories of isolation, 82
Alert category, 88
Enteric category, 90
Respiratory category, 92
Strict category, 94
Wound and skin category, 97
Reverse category, 99
Educational program, 101
Instructors, 101
Planning the program, 102
Program participants, 102
Introduction of speakers, 103
Checklist for program planners, 103
Methods of presenting the program, 104
Types of programs, 107
Evaluation, 111
Data collection, assimilation, and interpretation, 111
Purpose of reporting system, 112
Responsibility for collecting data, 112
Methods of collection, assimilation, and interpretation, 113
Problem solving, 120

4 Meeting the emotional needs of the isolation patient, 124

Pediatric patient in isolation, 125
Teen-ager in isolation, 126
Family, 126
Disseminating information, 127

5 Legal aspects of hospital-associated infections, 128

6 Interaction of health services and the hospital infection program, 132

American Hospital Association (AHA), 132
Center for Disease Control (CDC), 132
Public Health Service (PHS), 133
Public health nurse, 134
School nurse, 135
Interhospital infection control committee, 135
Organization, 135
Establishing guidelines, 136
Areas where standardization may be beneficial, 136
Function, 136

7   Nursing care plans for the isolation patient, 138

Meningitis, especially meningococcal—respiratory category precautions, 138
Tuberculosis—respiratory category precautions, 139
Typhoid fever—enteric category precautions, 140
Enteric disease (salmonellosis, shigellosis, and amebic dysentery)—enteric
    category precautions, 142
Draining wounds with airborne pathogens (coagulase-positive staphylococcus
    and beta hemolytic streptococcus, grade A)—wound and skin/respiratory
    category precautions, 143
Draining wounds with nonairborne pathogens (*Proteus, Escherichia coli,
    Pseudomonas)*—wound and skin category precautions, 144
Gas gangrene—wound and skin category precautions, 144
Infectious and serum hepatitis—enteric category precautions, 145
Encephalitis, 146
Chickenpox—respiratory category precautions, 148

Glossary, 149

CHAPTER ONE

Microorganisms and infection

Although health care professionals possess a background in the study of microorganisms and their relation to human disease, a brief review of the most familiar microorganisms should prove helpful in the development of an infection prevention and control program.

That man cannot live in a sterile environment for a long period of time without severe consequences was discovered over a century ago by Louis Pasteur (1822-1895) and his colleagues. The years between 1882 and 1910 have been described as the golden age of discovery. It was during this period that most of the disease-causing pathogenic organisms were identified, making it possible to prevent and control many infections and diseases.

Microbiology is a science that studies the nature, morphology, physicochemical composition, and reproduction of microscopic living things. Within its scope are the subspecialties of bacteriology (bacteria), virology (viruses), mycology (fungi), protozoology (protozoa), parasitology (parasites), and immunology.

BACTERIA

In this review emphasis is being placed on bacteria, since these organisms are the major contributors to infection and disease as they relate to the health facility environment.

Optimum conditions

Bacteria, like any living organism, need certain conditions for growth, reproduction, and maintenance of life. Several factors influence the well-being of bacteria.

1. *Growth cycle* (Fig. 1-1). Bacteria have a growth cycle, just as man has stages of life. A tube of fresh liquid medium, with an inoculum of x number of organisms, provides proper conditions for growth through several phases of the cycle.

    a. The *lag phase* represents a period of adaptability to the new environment so that new growth can be initiated.

    b. In the *exponential phase* new cell material is being produced, and the multiplication of new cells occurs at an exponential rate until the nutrients become exhausted or metabolic substances that inhibit growth are produced.

    c. In the *stationary phase* there is a reduction of growth to a point where a minimum number of cells are produced and a corresponding number of cells begin to die, so that the overall number of cells remain constant.

    d. During the *death phase* nutrients are exhausted and toxic metabolic waste products have accumulated; therefore growth declines. Cells die at an increasing rate until only a few cells remain viable.

The time of the cycle depends on the organism; some organisms undergo a complete growth cycle in a matter of hours whereas others may need several days.

2. *Temperature.* For each bacterial species there is a temperature at which the organism grows best. The largest group of bacteria are termed mesophiles (moderate temperature lovers). They include organisms that live in or attack the human body; their best growth occurs between 20° and 43° C. The psychrophilic (cold-loving) organisms grow best at temperatures below 15° C. Thermophiles (heat-loving organisms) grow at temperatures of 45° C. and over. For most pathogenic bacteria the optimal temperature is 35° to 37° C. Since organisms have the ability to grow in a wide range of temperatures, they may be found in any environment.

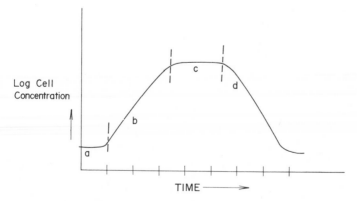

Fig. 1-1. Phases of bacterial growth cycle.

3. *pH.* pH is a concentration symbol that indicates the acidity or alkalinity of a solution. Most pathogenic organisms grow best in a solution with a neutral pH of 7. Few organisms grow in an acid pH under 5 or in an alkaline pH above 7.

4. *Oxygen requirements.* Microorganisms that can live and grow in the presence of free oxygen are called aerobes. Most pathogens will require some oxygen to survive and multiply. Those which thrive best or live only without oxygen are known as anaerobes. An organism preferring free oxygen but capable of growing in its absence is described as facultative. Microaerophilic organisms require only a small amount of oxygen for growth.

Morphology

Microorganisms differ in shape and size, and many of their names are derived from their appearance. Three basic shapes are generally recognized (Fig. 1-2): (1) coccic—spherical, (2) bacillary—rod-shaped, and (3) spiral—curved rods or spiral-shaped.

Cocci (from the Greek *kokkos,* meaning "berry") may be oval or elongated. The manner in which they divide and cling together aids in their identification. Cocci that group to form grapelike clusters are called *staphylococci;* those which form chains are known as *streptococci;* when found in pairs they are called *diplococci;* groups of fours are termed *tetrads;* and groups of eight or sixteen individual organisms may join together to form *cubes.*

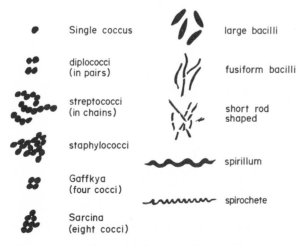

Fig. 1-2. Basic bacterial shapes and group formations.

Bacilli (from the Latin *bacillus,* meaning "a little stick or rod") are rod-shaped and may appear in many styles, such as short and fat, long and thin, or slightly curved. Those resembling cocci are named *coccobacilli.*

Spiral bacteria have a cylindrical shape. The *vibrios* are curved, resembling a comma. The *spirilla* are shaped like a corkscrew and are relatively rigid. The *spirochetes* are similar to the spirilla but differ in flexibility of body movements.

Reproduction

The process of typical bacterial reproduction is asexual by simple transverse division. The mature cell begins the cycle by constricting through the middle until it separates into two new organisms. Reproduction is species specific—like always begets like.

The rate of multiplication varies with the species and the conditions in which the organism grows. Under the best conditions the new cells may reach maturity and divide within a time span of 10 to 30 minutes.

Sporulation

The living bacterial cell is referred to as the vegetative cell. Under certain conditions this cell will change into a resistant body called a spore. When environmental conditions become favorable the spore covering breaks open, allowing the original cell to form. This is a protective mechanism rather than a reproductive process. The spore is capable of withstanding high temperatures for long periods of time, and special methods are required for its destruction. Not all bacteria are sporeformers, but the bacteria that cause tetanus, gas gangrene, botulism, and anthrax are always sporeformers.

Staining

Microorganisms are difficult to differentiate accurately, even under a microscope, unless they have been stained. In 1884, Danish histologist Hans Christian Gram developed the Gram stain procedure that is now used universally. Bacteria are classified as either positive or negative, depending on their stain reaction. Organisms that take up and retain the crystal violet stain will appear purplish under the microscope, and are known as grampositive. Some organisms that do not retain the crystal violet will absorb and retain the pink or red counterstain, safranin. These organisms are identified as gram-negative.

This method is not conducive to the identification of the spore. The dye penetrates only the bacteria but not the spore area, which remains clear, and is difficult to visualize if the surrouding areas are also colorless. Therefore, special differential stain techniques are required for spore visualization.

NORMAL FLORA

Normal flora are microorganisms in man or animals that assist the body in maintaining health equilibrium by preventing overgrowth of harmful bacteria. The term "normal flora" may be misleading, since normal in one person may be abnormal in another because of diet, climate, customs, race, and other factors. Within the individual's own body, characteristic features of the various body areas influence the type of organism that may be established. Different areas acquire different organisms as normal flora. Usually an equilibrium exists between the host and the normal flora. In order to survive, a new organism must adapt to the environment it has invaded.

Table 1. Location and type of normal body flora

BODY SITE	RESIDENT MICROBES
Mouth	Pigmented and nonpigmented micrococci (aerobic and anaerobic)
	Staphylococci
	Alpha hemolytic streptococci
	Beta hemolytic streptococci
	Microaerophilic and anaerobic streptococci
	Veillonella
	Vibrio
	Fusiform bacilli
	Borrelia
	Spirillum
	Treponema
	Gram-positive bacilli
	Gram-negative bacilli
	Candida
	Geotrichum
	Mycoplasma
	Actinomycetes
Throat	Nonhemolytic streptococci
	Neisseria
	Gram-negative bacilli such as:
	Pseudomonas
	Escherichia
	Proteus
	Citrobacter
	Klebsiella-Enterobacter-Serratia group
	Staphylococci
	Lactobacilli
	Corynebacterium
	Bacteroides
	Alphahemolytic streptococci

Continued.

Table 1. Location and type of normal body flora—cont'd

BODY SITE	RESIDENT MICROBES
Nasopharynx	*Diplococcus pneumoniae* *Corynebacterium* Alpha hemolytic streptococci Beta hemolytic streptococci *Haemophilus influenzae* *Neisseria*
Trachea Bronchi Lungs	Essentially sterile
Accessory nasal sinuses Mastoid sinuses	Essentially sterile
Stomach	Essentially sterile

Genitourinary tract	*Mycobacterium smegmatis*
	Gram-positive cocci
	    Alpha hemolytic streptocci
	    Nonhemolytic streptococci
	    Staphylococcus
	Corynebacterium
	Enterococci
	Lactobacillus
	Escherichia coli
	Yeasts

Intestinal tract	Alpha and beta hemolytic streptococci *Staphylococcus* *Corynebacterium* Klebsiella-Enterobacter-Serratia group *Escherichia coli* *Proteus* *Pseudomonas* *Neisseria* *Lactobacillus* *Clostridium* *Bacteroides* Other anaerobic species *Candida* *Aspergillus* *Penicillium* Enterococci

Mouth

There is a great variation in the number and type of organisms present in a healthy mouth. The large amounts of organic material present serve as nutrient material for a luxuriant population of organisms. The mouth of the newborn infant is not sterile at birth; it usually contains the same type of organisms that are present in the mother's vagina at that time. However, this original flora is gradually replaced by the organisms found in the infant's environment.

Throat

Very soon after birth, streptococci become the dominant flora. All types of bacteria are filtered from the air and inhaled through the nostrils. They may take up residence in the nasopharynx, trachea, and bronchi if they are not trapped in the mucous secretions of the nose and nasopharynx. Few organisms reach the trachea or bronchi, and those that do are usually eliminated by mechanical or immunologic means. If either of these mechanisms is not functioning, the organisms remain, multiply, and cause infection.

Nasopharynx

Some of the organisms residing in the nasopharynx are potential pathogens. The convalescent patient recovering from a specific infection and the healthy carrier harboring the organism are the reservoirs from which new clinical cases may arise. In the following example, normal flora in one area of the body causes disease in another part of the same body:

Alpha hemolytic streptococci are of no concern when found in the mouth of a healthy individual. However, if the individual has had rheumatic fever, it is possible for these bacteria to enter the bloodstream through the gums after tooth extraction and lodge on the heart valves, producing a subacute bacterial endocarditis.

Trachea, bronchi, lungs, and accessory nasal and mastoid sinuses

The trachea, bronchi, lungs, and accessory nasal and mastoid sinuses are essentially sterile areas in the healthy individual.

Stomach

Although many organisms reach the stomach from the salivary and nasopharyngeal secretions, the healthy stomach has no natural flora. Organisms secreted into the stomach are usually killed by the high acidity or the digestive enzymes of the gastric juices. In some cases, organisms pass so rapidly from the stomach to the intestinal tract that they are not destroyed in this area. In abnormal conditions of the stomach (carcinoma or obstruction) food is retained and begins to demonstrate a characteristic flora of its own. These organisms are usually identified as *Sarcina,* yeast, and a gram-positive organism known as the Boas-Oppler bacillus *(Lactobacillus acidophilus).*

Duodenum

The duodenum is usually sterile unless an infection is present in the gallbladder.

Below the duodenum

At birth the entire tract is sterile. The anaerobic lactobacilli are the first organisms populating the area. The microorganisms increase progressively in number as they proceed through the intestinal tract, with the maximum number occurring in the colon. Under certain conditions the resident flora in the intestinal tract may be responsible for disease. The genus *Bacteroides,* which normally resides in the large intestine, may produce a serious infection if it leaves its normal habitat and is introduced into the peritoneal cavity or into an open wound. *Escherichia coli* and *Proteus* species are nonpathogenic in the bowel area, but if they enter an obstructed urinary tract or a wound, an infection will result.

The "Turista" that plagues so many travelers may very well be due to an *Escherichia coli* serotype that is not normally carried by the patient but was picked up from a human contact.

During hot weather children often do not eat properly nor drink enough fluids. This permits large amounts of undigested foods to reach the small intestine, where it is met by the invading *Escherichia coli* from the large bowel area. The organic acids produced by this organism irritate the gut, resulting in a diarrhea. Thus the so-called "summer diarrhea" of children may be due to a spontaneous alteration of normal flora in the intestinal tract.

Routine use of broad-spectrum antibiotics has a profound effect on normal intestinal flora. If enough large doses of antibiotics are given, suppression of the gram-positive organisms may result, leading to an overgrowth of *Escherichia coli, Enterobacter* species, *Proteus* species, and *Pseudomonas aeruginosa.* These organisms may now invade the bloodstream and produce a bacteremia and possibly a septicemia that may lead to death. Dosage of antibiotics may be large enough to suppress both gram-positive and gram-negative organisms, leading to disease caused by an overgrowth of *Candida albicans* or some other opportunistic fungus. On occasion all organisms may be destroyed and a resistant strain may develop. A prime example is enteritis caused by *Staphylococcus aureus.* This organism may be the predominant organism left in the intestine after massive doses of antibiotics have been given; under these conditions it will produce a disease state.

Sterilization of the intestinal tract may interfere with the production of the B-complex vitamins and of vitamin K. Some of these vitamins are not produced by the body but are by-products of bacterial metabolism in the intestinal tract. The lack of vitamin K can cause a bleeding syndrome.

Genitourinary tract

The kidneys, ureters, and bladder area are normally sterile, although some organisms may be present in the female urethra. A wide variety of saprophytes may be isolated in both males and females. The type of flora present will vary with the age of the individual.

Skin

The skin is primarily considered a single site, but its bacterial population varies in the different anatomic regions: for example, the flora of the facial area reflects that of the nasopharynx, whereas the bacteria of the lower intestinal tract influence the type of flora of the perineal area. Although vigorous scrubbing of the skin with soap, water, or disinfectant (as in a surgical prep scrub) will aid in the temporary removal of most of the skin's surface bacteria, organisms in hair follicles and sweat glands will soon repopulate the skin surface.

Other areas

Human milk contains large numbers of bacteria, but no problems will ensue unless some of them are pathogenic. The bloodstream, cerebrospinal fluid, and lymph nodes are all sterile; therefore, any organism isolated from these areas would indicate an infectious process.

PATHOGENS

Normal flora provides the body with equilibrium that promotes health and prevents disease. When this balance is destroyed by overgrowth of any one organism or by invasion of pathogens, disease or infection ensues.

Just as a healthy body has built-in substances such as mucus and acid to protect itself against harmful invasion, pathogens also have safeguards. Thus many species of bacteria yield poisonous matter called *toxins*.

Exotoxins diffuse into the surrounding body medium to cause such diseases as diphtheria, tetanus, gas gangrene, and botulism. These toxins are stimulated generally by gram-positive bacteria. They have an affinity for the tissues of nerves, as in tetanus, or kidney and heart muscles, as in diphtheria. The toxin can easily be neutralized by a specific antitoxin. If the disease is acute, antitoxins or hyperimmune serums are available.

Endotoxins are lipopolysaccharides produced by gram-negative organisms. When these bacterial cells are destroyed, a weak toxin is released.

Endotoxins may be the cause of typhoid fever, salmonellosis, cholera, brucellosis, or gram-negative shock.

Staphylococci, streptococci, and other organisms produce a substance known as a *lysin,* which hemolyzes animal red blood cells. These substances are proteins and can induce the formation of antibodies in the body against themselves. Other organisms produce a *leukocidin,* which may destroy the polymorphonuclear neutrophil (PMN) leukocytes in the blood. These blood cells are essential to the body's defense mechanism.

Staphylococcus aureus produces a *coagulase* capable of clotting plasma, which may result in emboli, sometimes seen in severe infections. Microorganisms can also produce *kinases,* which liquefy clots. In an inflammation area where the plasma has clotted to seal off the area, kinase can penetrate the clot, causing it to dissolve and to allow the organisms entrapped in the sealed-off section to spread to other parts of the body.

Hyaluronidase, secreted by certain streptococci or pneumonococci, produces a substance that facilitates tissue penetration by bacteria. It destroys hyaluronic acid, which acts as a cement to hold tissue cells intact.

Capsules—the capsular material surrounding *Haemophilus influenzae* or *Diplococcus pneumoniae*—act as a protective agent for the organism and make bacterial cell destruction more difficult.

The indiscriminate use of *antibiotics* may cause microbial changes through mutation and result in bacteria with increased drug resistance. Strains of bacteria have emerged that are more and more resistant to one antibiotic or to closely related groups of antibiotics. Resistance is usually followed by a clinical disease that has been inadequately treated or overtreated.

EPIDEMIOLOGY OF INFECTION

Epidemiology is the study of the occurrence and distribution of disease as it is prevalent in man. It is based on the history of disease as known by experts or experienced by the populace; frequency and modes of development of disease in its relationship to climatic conditions; habits of the populace and their attitudes toward disease; and the specific means used for prevention and control.

Epidemic is a term applied to the occurrence of a disease in many people at the same time or in rapid succession; in one or more persons in an area where the disease had not previously been recognized; or in one or more persons where the disease, such as smallpox, had not been reported in at least ten years. If a disease is epidemic at the same time in many different parts of the world, it is said to be *pandemic.* An *endemic* disease is one that is generally present in a given locality in a certain number of the population. Most infectious diseases are endemic in some locality and do

not usually become epidemic, since the infectious agent is of ordinary virulence and most people in the environment have immunity. However, an
endemic disease may become epidemic if a considerable number of persons lack immunity or if the infectious agent suddenly becomes more
virulent than usual.

The development of any infectious disease is dependent on a sequence
of factors often referred to as a cycle (Fig. 1-3). Breaking this cycle is
vital in the prevention and control of infection. The factors involved in
this infectious process are as follows:

1. The microbial or infectious agent that lives and multiplies
2. The source or reservoir in which it develops
3. Its escape through the portal of exit
4. Its transmission by various modes
5. Its entry into the new source through the appropiate portal of entry

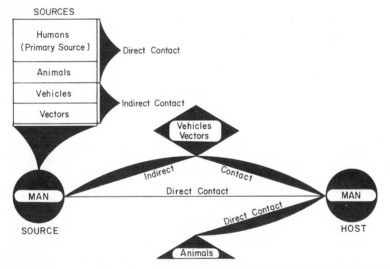

SOURCES				
HUMANS	ANIMALS	SOCIAL CONTACT	VEHICLES	VECTORS
Patients	Cats	Hands	Inanimate	Pigeons
Visitors	Dogs	Kissing	— Food	Mosquitos
Personnel	Rodents	Sexual Intercourse	— Water	Flies
Medical Staff		Coughing	— Drugs	Ticks
		Sneezing	— Blood	Lice
			— Soil	Fleas
			— Air	
			— Fomites	

Fig. 1-3. Elements of the spread of disease in the hospital environment.

6. Its maturation and multiplication in the new source (a susceptible host)

The etiologic or infectious agent must be sufficiently virulent to produce a disease state in man. Either the organism's secretions or excretions or the organism itself must invade the cell. Once this happens, destruction of the cell or multiplication of the organism or both occur. Some of the organisms capable of producing diseases are bacteria, protozoa, rickettsiae, fungi, viruses, and helminths. Endogenous organisms are those that are part of the normal flora or those potentially virulent organisms already residing in the host that, given the right circumstances, are capable of producing disease (for example, *Escherichia coli* in a postsurgical wound after a perineal resection). Other microorganisms that invade from outside the host are described as exogenous (for example, *Corynebacterium diphtheriae*).

The source, or reservoir, is the environment, either human, animal, or inanimate, in which the organism lives and multiplies. The human source in the hospital involves the entire hospital population—patients, personnel, visitors, and others who enter the hospital environment for any reason.

Humans who act as sources for specific disease organisms may either (1) have a typical case, (2) have a mild, atypical, or unrecognized case, (3) have a latent or dormant case, or (4) be a carrier.

The individual who is suffering from a *typical* communicable disease will show visible symptoms and some clinical evidence, and will usually be able to recognize the incubation exposure time.

Mild and *atypical* cases occur frequently. The individual may be infected with virulent organisms, but the symptoms may be so slight that the disease goes unrecognized and therefore unreported to the health authorities.

In some infections, such as tuberculosis, the organism can remain *latent* or *dormant* for years. Although the organism is still present in the body, there are no symptoms until the presence of the organism is manifested later, at a time when the host's body resistance is lowered.

The most "silent" of the human sources is the healthy *carrier,* who harbors disease-producing organisms in his body but has not developed symptoms of the illness at any time. *Convalescent carriers* (such as patients with hepatitis) remain a source of infection long after the major symptoms have disappeared. In some cases they may remain carriers for the rest of their lives.

Common *inanimate* sources are soil, air, food, water, milk, feces, and fomites. The organisms that cause tetanus and gas gangrene may be deposited in the soil through the feces of animals or men and survive for long periods of time.

Organisms grow rapidly in such media as *food* and *milk* unless they are destroyed by heat or retarded by cold. *Fomites* such as soiled bed linen, bedpans, emesis basins, and freshly contaminated instruments or equipment are excellent sources in which pathogenic organisms may live and multiply until they can be transmitted to a susceptible host.

Mode of transmission is the transfer of infective organisms from one host, or source, to another. The relative danger of spread depends on a ability of the organism to survive outside the reservoir. Organisms with a low survival rate outside the reservoir are commonly transmitted through personal contact with infected hosts.

Direct transfer of the organisms may be made through actual physical contact, as in venereal disease transmission through kissing or sexual intercourse, which permits body contact with secretions that are harboring the infective organisms.

Some organisms with a short survival time may be directly transmitted through infectious *droplets* that are coughed or sneezed within close range of a susceptible host. This is especially true in patients with meningitis (meningococcal). These organisms, which are protected from the environment by means of a mucous coating, or by their spore form, can remain viable for long periods of time; for example, *M. tuberculosis* in sputum will be infectious for several weeks.

Contaminated hands are probably the most important medium of transmission, especially in regard to the fecal-oral route in the spread of enteric diseases (for example, salmonellosis and hepatitis).

The mode of transmission through *indirect contact* involves an intermediary, on which the infective organism persists outside the reservoir until it is transferred to another host. Such intermediaries are known as *vehicles* and *vectors*.

A *vehicle* may be water (typhoid), milk (bacillary dysentery and tuberculosis), air (respiratory infections), or fomites. *Fomites* are inanimate objects such as drinking glasses, silverware, and toilet articles that have been contaminated by the infected patient or visitor. The organisms may remain alive on these fomites and be transmitted to the mouth or nose by the hands; by eating with the contaminated silverware; or by drinking from the contaminated glass.

Vectors are mainly arthropods that transmit pathogenic organisms by either mechanical or biologic means. The organisms transmitted are usually species specific—mosquitoes carry yellow fever, ticks transmit Rocky Mountain spotted fever, and flies transfer the typhoid bacillus. In *mechanical* transmission, the infected organism may adhere to the insect's body and be carried from place to place. For example, flies may carry organisms from excreta to food, causing dysentery, typhoid fever, or cholera. *Biologic* transmission takes place when the insect (mosquito, louse, tick) acts as an intermediate host by biting an infected host, ingesting the organism, harboring it for a time, and then finally transmitting the infective organism through biting another host, or through its feces.

The *portal of entry* is usually the same as the portal of exit: the nose, mouth, eyes, ears, genitals, broken skin, lesions, wounds, urinary or intestinal tracts, or, before birth, the placenta.

The *host* must be susceptible before the organism is able to cause an infection or disease. The body's resistance may be lowered through the following factors:

1. Age (the very young or the very old)
2. Drugs (frequent or continuous use of antibiotics, cortisone, or steroids)
3. Immunosuppressive drugs (frequently used in cancer or in organ transplants)
4. Heavy irradiation (which causes a breakdown in the body tissue and depresses the immune response)
5. Malnutrition
6. Chronic diseases (uremia, diabetes, cancer, nephrosis, leukemia)
7. Shock (which lowers the body's resistance due to the frequent metabolic interference of the disease and the eventual breakdown of important body functions)

BODY'S NATURAL DEFENSES

A healthy body is provided with normal defenses and has the ability to fight the invading organism.

Unbroken skin is the body's first line of defense. It offers excellent protection since, with few exceptions, organisms cannot pass through it. Many of the skin's secretions are bactericidal and actually kill the organism. A bacteriostatic agent only inhibits multiplication of the bacterium but does not kill. If the skin is injured or punctured even microscopically, microorganisms may enter underlying tissues. Neglect of skin injuries may lead to serious inflammation with pus formation, especially if the injured area comes in contact with infectious material. When skin is badly damaged by fire or is burned by chemicals, it can no longer function in the normal manner since water cannot escape properly from the body. The skin is then moist and warm and contains a number of nutrients that produce an environment in which bacteria can readily grow.

The *conjunctiva* is protected by the motion of the eyelids and by the constant washing of the tears. This process carries microorganisms down to the nose and eliminates them in this fashion. Tears contain a secretion called lysozyme, which may be bactericidal. Organisms can enter via the eye and, in spite of its protective structure, cause such diseases as pneumo-coccal conjunctivitis or ophthalmic gonorrhea.

The *lungs* are protected by the complex arrangement of the nasal passages with the moist membranes and cilia. Dust, bacteria, and other particles adhere to the membrane secretions and are expelled through sneezing or some other mechanical means. Lower in the respiratory tract, foreign material may be expelled by coughing and the upward movement of particular matter by the cilia. If the bacteria in this area are pathogenic, the normal defense mechanisms may not be capable of preventing invasion.

The acidic nature of the gastric juices will kill some organisms. The *gastrointestinal tract* also gains some protection from the bile secretions that enter the upper portion of the small intestines. The bile will destroy many organisms that enter from the stomach. Another defense mechanism is the ingestion and digestion of bacteria by phagocytes (polymorphonu-clear leukocytes and monocytes).

The *genitourinary system* is afforded a degree of protection by its rather thick layer of cells, the acidic nature of the area, and the mucous secretions. None of these factors prevent invasion by *Neisseria gonorrhoeae, Treponema pallidum,* and the beta hemolytic streptococci.

Certain *leukocytes* and *tissue cells* make up a very important defense mechanism for the body. Some of the white blood cells act as "scavengers" or "police" in the blood. Any foreign particles such as bacteria or dead tissue cells that enter blood or tissue are surrounded and engulfed by these cells (process of phagocytosis).

Chemical protection against disease is provided by certain substances in the blood. Properdin, one such substance, is a protein that may be related to the complement system. The two together may serve as protection against viruses and bacteria. When viruses are present in tissue cells, the cells are stimulated to produce *interferon,* a protein that *kills* viruses. This is a natural defense mechanism useful in terminating viral infections.

Inflammation is a very important process that is necessary for body protection. It is a defensive response of living tissue to any agent that irritates or injures this tissue. The four cardinal signs of inflammation are redness, swelling, heat, and pain. Redness and heat, caused by the dilation of blood vessels, increases the blood flow in the involved area. At the laceration site a blood clot forms a plug to prevent the organism's entrance into the general circulation system. In the inflammatory process, exudate and cells seep from the dilated vessels into the surrounding tissue. This mass of cells (erythrocytes and leukocytes) liberates enzymes that liquefy the cells to form pus. Gradually other blood substances are released, fibrin is formed, and a wall results to protect the body from the inflammatory site. If pus formation is not evacuated from the injured site by incision or drainage, an abscess, from which infectious material will travel along muscle sheaths or through the body sinuses to infect more areas, may result. However, if incision and drainage of the abscess is adequate, new tissue granulations begin to grow inward and upward until a scar is formed.

Immunity is the resistance of the body to infection or disease. It is a term usually applied to protection of the individual against the invasion of a pathogenic microorganism. Certain races of people are said to have natural immunity against specific diseases, possibly due to generations of built-up resistance.

Newborn infants possess a temporary protection against some diseases until they are 3 or 4 months old, through antibodies supplied directly from the mother's bloodstream. This immunity is described as *passive* since the person himself did not produce the antibody. *Active* immunity may be *acquired* naturally, through recovery from a communicable disease, or artificially, through *immunization*. The introduction of foreign protein substances (antigens in the form of vaccines) into the bloodstream stimulates specialized cells in the body to produce a protective *antibody*. The reaction of the *antigen-antibodies* provides the body with defense against specific infections and diseases. These antigens can be killed, attenuated, or live microbes.

The duration of immunity acquired by *vaccination* varies with the antigen used, the dosage, and the age and health of the individual.

By *interrupting one sequence* of the infectious process, diseases may be prevented or controlled. This is the purpose of all health measures such as pasteurization, sterilization, sanitation, isolation, and immunization.

The epidemiology of a particular disease and its prevalence in man determines the basis for specific standards of prevention and control of infection and disease in the hospital. Characteristics that distinguish infections in the hospital as either community or hospital associated, as well as a method of classification of types, must be determined by the infection control committee. The following discussion is a guide to defining and classifying infections and diseases that are found in and about the hospital environment.

COMMUNITY- AND HOSPITAL-ASSOCIATED INFECTIONS

Community-associated infections are those found in patients who enter the hospital with a known or incubating infection. A patient admitted with an infection has the ability to spread it to susceptible persons in a hospital setting; therefore community-associated infections are relevant to the general trend of hospital-associated infections. The *nosocomial,* or *hospital-associated, infection* is an infection that appears to have developed during hospitalization or is not known to have been incubating at the time of admission. The definition of nosocomial infection is quite broad since its determination is essentially a matter of symptoms supported by clinical judgment, and many of the infections are borderline. Thus nosocomial infections include potentially preventable infections as well as some infections that may be regarded as inevitable.

Community-associated infections are easily identified, since the presence of an infection at the time of admission is usually established. Hospital-associated infections are more difficult to define.

If the physician indicates in the chart that a nosocomial infection is or has been present, then the information is recorded unequivocally as an infection, whether or not additional supporting data are present in the chart. In the absence of such specific information, the examiner must then make a judgment as to whether the chart reviewed reveals an infection. . . . There must be a high degree of certainty as to when the clinical manifestations of the infections in question had their onset.*

Classification of infections†

For comparison and review, infections in the hospital are usually best classified by five types: respiratory, urinary tract, gastrointestinal, wound and skin, and others.

Respiratory infections include both upper and lower respiratory infections. Signs and symptoms vary widely and depend on the sites involved.

Urinary tract infection determination is usually based on bacterial colony count in urine (usually >100,000 organisms per milliliter) and a positive or negative urine culture before administration of antibiotics.

Gastrointestinal infections are generally based on clinical evidence of stool specimens and the known incubation period for the pathogen (for example, salmonella or shigella).

Wound and skin infections will include any purulent drainage from a surgical site and in addition, abscesses; they are usually confirmed by cultures of fluid aspirates.

Others is a classification used for any infection that is not compatible with distinct classifications. It includes septicemias; infections from catheter tips or filters or from intravenous needles; infection indicated by fever of undetermined origin; communicable diseases such as hepatitis and viral exanthems; and vaginal infections involving, for example, lochia and pelvic infection disease (PID).

Classification depends mainly on site, and care should be taken to

---

*From Outline for surveillance and control of nosocomial infections, Atlanta, 1970, Center for Disease Control.
†Based on Outline for surveillance and control of nosocomial infections, Atlanta, 1970, Center for Disease Control.

report correctly where the infection developed (tracheal infections could be classified as either wound (site of surgery), respiratory (secretion), or other (equipment or tracheotomy tube).

REFERENCES

Davis, B. D., Delbecco, R., Eisen, H. N., Ginsberg, H. S., and Wood, W. B.: Microbiology, New York, 1967, Hoeber Medical Division, Harper & Row, Publishers.

Isenberg, H. D.: Indigenous and pathogenic microorganisms of man. In Manual of clinical microbiology, Bethesda, Md., 1970, American Society for Microbiology.

Rosebury, T.: Microorganisms indigenous to man, New York, 1962, McGraw-Hill Book Co.

Smith, A. L.: Microbiology and pathology, ed. 10, St. Louis, 1972, The C. V. Mosby Co.

CHAPTER TWO

Infection control structure and organization

INFECTION CONTROL COMMITTEE

In 1958 the Joint Commission on Accreditation of Hospitals (JCAH) and the American Hospital Association issued recommendations on setting up an infection control committee, charged with the responsibility of investigation, control, and prevention of infections within hospitals. Membership and functions of the committee were listed. Experience has proved the soundness of these recommendations. The revised version is as follows:

In order to provide guidelines for hospitals in the fulfillment of these responsibilities, the Committee on Infection Within Hospitals of the American Hospital Association developed and published the following recommendations:

All hospitals should establish Committees on Infection, to devote particular attention to infections that are acquired in hospitals so they may be reduced to the lowest possible minimum.

1. It is suggested that the Committee on Infection include, where possible, a bacteriologist, a pediatrician, a surgeon, an internist, a nurse, and a hospital administrator. The local health officer should be urged to serve as a consultant to the committee. The committee should report periodically to the executive committee of the medical staff.

2. The functions of the Committee on Infection should include at least the following:

   a. Establish a system of reporting infection among patients and personnel, such a system being essential to a proper understanding of infection acquired in hospitals. The committee should have access to all reports of infection anywhere in the hospital.

   b. Keep records of infections as a basis for the study of their sources and for recommendations regarding remedial measures.

   c. Distinguish to the best of its ability between infection acquired in the hospital and that acquired outside.

   d. Review the hospital's bacteriological services to make sure that such services are of high quality and are accessible either in the hospital itself or in an outside laboratory. Bacteriophage typing, if not available in the hospital, may be sought as needed through official local and state health agencies.

   e. Review aseptic techniques employed in operating rooms, delivery rooms, nurseries, and in the treatment of all patients with infections, and, if indicated, recommend methods to improve these techniques and their enforcement.

   f. Make vigorous efforts to reduce to the minimum consistent with adequate patient care:

     (1) Use of antibiotics, especially as "prophylaxis" in clean, elective surgery.

     (2) Treatment with adrenocortical steroids.

   g. Undertake an educational program to convince medical staff and hospital employees of the importance of reporting to responsible authorities when they have skin infections, boils, acute upper respiratory infections, and the like.

   h. Establish techniques for discovering infections which do not become manifest until after discharge from the hospital, it being known that such infections are often overlooked because they may not be apparent until several weeks after the patient has left the hospital. Two approaches to discovering such infections are suggested:

     (1) An attempt to trace the source of any infection with which a patient may be admitted. For example, if an infant is admitted with staphylococcal pneumonia, or a recently delivered mother with mastitis, the hospital where delivery occurred should be informed of the infection so that it can seek possible sources of infection.

     (2) Periodic telephone polls on a random sample of discharged patients (particularly recently delivered mothers, newborns, and postoperative patients) to ascertain their state of health and, in case of an indication of infection, to follow it up. Such surveys have proven quite simple and quite valuable. A detailed account of the method is given by Ravenholt and others in the October 1956 issue of the *American Journal of Public Health*."*

The responsibility for establishing the hospital's infection control committee will depend on the individual hospital's line of authority. The medical staff advisory committee, consisting of the organized medical staff's executive committee and selected members, is usually given this duty.

---

*From Infection control in the hospital, rev. ed., Chicago, 1970, American Hospital Association, pp. 15 and 16.

The members of the committee are responsible to the hospital's board of trustees for the professional care of the patient and collaborate with the administrator on decisions concerning standards of patient care.

One person is designated as the hospital epidemiologist or chairman of the infection control committee. He is usually appointed by the hospital's chief of staff and is often the bacteriologist or pathologist, or an active member of the medical staff. To qualify, the chairman should have a knowledge of epidemiology and professional stature that will command the respect of his colleagues.

Committee membership

The selection and composition of the committee will vary with the individual hospital. In some hospitals the chairman prepares a list of representatives from the various departments and specialties and submits it to the chief of staff for approval.

A well-organized committee membership will include departmental infection control officers who are physicians representing the major clinical departments (medical, surgical, obstetrics-gynecology, nursery, pediatrics); a pathologist; representatives from personnel health services (physician or health nurse), the nursing service, environmental services, dietary service, pharmacy, central service, respiratory therapy, and the local health department; and the infection control nurse (nurse epidemiologist). Some members may be designated as ex-officio.

Functions

The *chairman* assumes general supervision of the infection control program in the hospital and advises the administration on problems of prevention, detection, and control of infectious diseases. Under his direction, the committee establishes a system of reporting infections among patients and personnel, and keeps the medical staff and hospital employees currently informed in matters of infection control. In addition to general supervision of the infection control program, the chairman may supervise and direct the nurse epidemiologist, initiate action in matters of infection control as established by the infection control committee, and determine temporary criteria or regulations where none exist. However, such action should be subject to prompt review by the infection control committee. He should have free access to patients' records and the authority to consult with a patient's physician if necessary.

The infection control *departmental officers* should be responsible for establishing and implementing the infection control policies and procedures within their respective departments, and should work closely with the nurse epidemiologist. Prompt and accurate reporting of actual or potential sources of contagion within the department should be made to the departmental officer by personnel of his department.

Committee *representatives* of hospital areas should be consulted and authorized to take immediate action on infection control problems arising in their area. The representatives will also work closely with the nurse epidemiologist.

Any interdepartmental conflicts should be handled by the chairman of the committee.

It is essential to the success of the committee and the infection control program that a good working relationship exists between the nurse epidemiologist and the chairman. The nurse epidemiologist is responsible for detecting and recording nosocomial infections on a systematic and current basis, but the infection control committee must provide definitions of nosocomial infections that are workable and consistent. The committee is also responsible for establishing and maintaining a continuing educational program for all hospital personnel in the prevention and control of infections.

ROLE OF THE NURSE EPIDEMIOLOGIST

A surveillance program is essential to prevention and control of infections in hospitals. In many instances, physicians, health officers, microbiologists, nursing service supervisors, and others trained in allied fields serve as part-time hospital epidemiologists. Hospital department heads are required to report to the infection control committee, and the part-time surveillance officer assembles the information and presents it in the form of a monthly report to the infection control committee. It has been estimated that a bare minimum of 20 hours of work per week is usually required for surveillance in a 250-bed hospital.* The rise in incidence of hospital-associated infections points up the growing need for a full-time surveillance officer.

The nurse's role as a specialist in health care facilities has already been expanded in several areas. One vital area of nurse specialization is in the field of surveillance. The nurse is involved in direct patient care, provides continuous professional supervision, and can more readily adapt these principles to prevention and control of diseases and infections to achieve uniformity in the infection program. It is essential that one person be authorized to supervise the hospital program daily. Since the chairman of the committee and the committee members have work commitments in addition to the committee work, an infection control nurse or a nurse epidemiologist should be appointed.

---

*Outline for surveillance and control of nosocomial infections, Atlanta, 1970, Center for Disease Control.

Qualifications

The nurse epidemiologist should have a bachelor of science in nursing degree or, preferably, a bachelor of science degree in microbiology or a science relating to the field, as well as a working knowledge of statistics. A public health background in disease symptom etiology, and in host, agent, and environment interaction is an excellent accouterment to surveillance qualifications. Education in infection prevention and control is essential to program planning, and schedules of available courses may be obtained from the Center for Disease Control, Atlanta, Georgia.

In addition to a workable knowledge of prevention and control of infections, the nurse epidemiologist should possess an abundance of tact, patience, and stamina.

Functions

The most immediate function of the nurse epidemiologist is to assist the infection control committee in the establishment of a surveillance

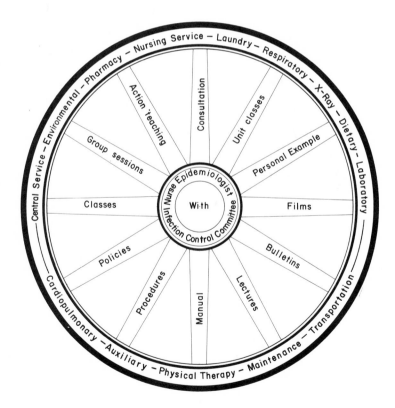

Fig. 2-1. Interdepartmental flow of information.

system. Once such a system is established, the efforts of the nurse epidemiologist are directed toward actively involving all the departments of the hospital into the program and in maintaining an efficient unified system. This goal is accomplished through the flow of information to all departments of the hospital, where it is assimilated into the individual departmental procedures and returned, through practice, to become a part of the unified whole. (See Fig. 2-1.)

The functions of the nurse epidemiologist extend beyond establishing and maintaining the surveillance program. The professional training and skills of this specialist are utilized in selecting the correct approach in meeting the emotional needs of the isolation patient; creating an awareness of the legal aspects of hospital-associated infections; stimulating a close working relationship with community agencies; and assisting in the formulation of nursing care plans.

CHAPTER THREE

Developing the surveillance program

Surveillance programs will vary among hospitals since they are determined by the physical environment and facilities, and by the population, which consists of patients, personnel, medical staff, visitors, and volunteers. However, the basics remain the same. No infection prevention and control program, regardless of how well it is conceived, can effectively function without the personal involvement of every individual. The total program should contain the following:

1. Role of the nurse and physician
2. A personnel health service program
3. Policies and procedures for both prevention and control
4. Categories of isolation, with precautions pertaining to each
5. Education program for the hospital population
6. Data collection, assimilation, and interpretation

ROLE OF THE NURSE AND PHYSICIAN

Nurses are expected to know and perform all functions necessary to the total care of the patient, and this is especially true with the infectious patient. In addition to caring for the patient, the nurse must know how to protect others from contracting the disease and how to avoid contracting the disease herself. The nurse is also responsible for disseminating prevention and control information to personnel, patients, their families, and visitors.

The physician is responsible for accurately diagnosing the patient's need for isolation. He must protect his patient from infectious patients and the hospital personnel from his infected patient. He must work closely with the nurse in medical asepsis and be aware of new developments in infection control. The physician plays an important role in the event of a hospital epidemic, since it affects his patient. More immediate is his responsibility of serving as an example to hospital personnel in strict adherence to the prevention and control rules and regulations, especially frequent handwashing.

PERSONNEL HEALTH SERVICE PROGRAM

Health facilities personnel play a major role in the prevention and control of infections since they have a relationship with both patient and public. Every reasonable effort should be made to cultivate a safe and healthful working environment for the personnel. This goal may be accomplished in part by an effective personnel health service program.

The scope of the health service program will vary according to the health facility as to size, number of employees, and available funds. An important consideration in a good health program is its establishment as a separate functioning unit under professional supervision. However, all facilities should provide some basic health services to protect the employee from intramural infections and prevent spread of infection from employees to patients. Emphasis should be placed on motivation of the individual to accept responsibility for his own health.

Preemployment examination

Health facilities with an established employee health service clinic usually prefer to conduct their own preemployment examinations. In many instances employees are responsible for this examination by their own private physician.

Such an examination should include a history, physical examination, chest x-ray examination, blood serology test, tuberculosis skin test, and stool culture of personnel working in special areas such as the dietary service and the nursery. A Papanicolaou test and breast cancer detection are also essential to a good preventive personnel health program.

Immunizations

Recommended immunizations that should be made available to personnel are diphtheria, tetanus, influenza, typhoid, smallpox, measles, and poliomyelitis, as well as others pertinent to the geographic area.

Follow-up

Periodic physicals assure the employee of good health and discover health problems that may require treatment. Chest x-ray examinations, Papanicolaou tests, and breast cancer detection should be scheduled yearly. Stool and blood cultures should be scheduled on a six-month basis for personnel employed in high-risk areas. There should be periodic monitoring and blood tests of personnel who work in radiology and in nuclear medicine. Immunization boosters are important and should be made available at all times.

Other services

1. Employee examinations or tests should be made for any suspected infection or exposure to infection or contagious disease; treatment should be instituted if indicated.

2. First-aid or palliative treatment should be given to enable the employee to complete his current work shift.

3. Emergency care should be provided for injuries on the job, until the employee may be referred to his own physician.

4. Continuing education of good health practices, both at work and at home, should be made available. This education may also include classes in first aid, nutrition, or hazardous job safety. Health posters that caution about the spread of infection through coughing or sneezing and the dangers of smoking are good reminders. Booklets or films on diabetes detection, cancer detection, and personnel hygiene are readily available and should be utilized.

5. Counseling for handicapped personnel should be provided in order to place them in positions compatible with their performance. Employees should also be encouraged to secure counseling for emotional problems, dietary needs or chronic conditions such as high blood pressure.

6. For convenience, medical injections may be given to the hospital personnel in the clinic, if authorization is obtained from their private physicians. Prescription drugs should be sold to employees on a percentage discount basis.

7. Electrocardiograms should be made available to any employee, especially those over the age of 40 years.

8. Extracurricular activities conducive to good health, such as swimming, physical culture, weight control groups, bowling, golfing, or tennis teams, might be sponsored by the health facility.

9. In the nursery, the labor and delivery rooms, and pediatrics, all women employees of childbearing age should be tested for protection against rubella. Those with low titers should not work in these areas.

10. All employees should be encouraged to report an illness and not be penalized with loss of pay. Control of excessive time loss may be necessary by requiring the ill employee to call the health clinic when he cannot report for work and to report to the clinic before returning to work.

Health service nurse

The health service nurse has direct charge of the employee service program. It is her responsibility to schedule examinations, investigate health problems, and provide the immunizations that have been authorized by the hospital. She works closely with the nurse epidemiologist and is immediately alerted to any infectious problem.

Records

Complete health records should be confidentially filed in the clinic. There should be one for each employee in the hospital.

Personnel health services will promote the incentive to better work performance of the employee. It often reduces absenteeism, insurance costs, and employee turnover. A healthy employee is "money in the bank" for both employer and employee.

POLICIES AND PROCEDURES FOR PREVENTION AND CONTROL

Policies and procedures should be established for the hospital population, without exception. It is the responsibility of each department to participate in a program of continuing education to ensure proper understanding and application of each policy and procedure while providing for the physical and emotional well-being of the patient and his family.

Policies and procedures govern the standards of care and determine to a large extent the methods of preventing cross infection in the hospital, and indirectly in the community. They are usually established through the infection control committee, which is assisted by the nurse epidemiologist and representatives from each department of the hospital, and approved by the medical advisory board.

Although there may be overlapping of prevention and control measures, there are definite basics relating to each. *Prevention* relates to *eliminating* the occurrence of a disease or infection; *control* pertains to *restricting* the spread of existing diseases or infections.

A *manual* is a valuable tool for personnel in all hospital departments; its scope is determined by the complexities of the facility. Its contents should be as complete as possible.

A *policy* is a broadly stated governing principle that usually remains constant. A *procedure* is the method or steps taken to fulfill this policy; it will probably require frequent revision to keep abreast of changes. Although the elements of both are interrelated, they should not be combined but should be parallel—a procedure for every policy. Many policies may be so factual that detailed procedures are unnecessary. The policies should be included in the manual according to the planned arrangement.

Procedures should be written in a logical, orderly sequence, and those persons who thoroughly understand the subject should contribute to the content. Personnel from specialty areas should be consulted as necessary.

It should not be assumed that hospital staff or personnel are well versed in this special field; even the well-informed require refresher courses occasionally. The manual will also be utilized to promote efficiency and a feeling of security for nonprofessional personnel. To provide all possible assistance to its intended readers, the format of the manual should be basically uniform, its terminology simple, and all ideas expressed positively.

A good index, constant revision of existing procedures, and the addition of new procedures when indicated will promote frequent use of the manual. The purpose, equipment to be used, and any general comments should preface each procedure. The policies and procedures suggested here may be adapted to meet the requirements of the individual hospital and guide the administrative staff in formulating a surveillance system.

Prevention policies and procedures

Basic prevention policies and procedures are essential in minimizing the possibility of infection and providing a superior and safe hospital environment. They are established by the Joint Commission on the Accreditation of Hospitals for all departments of the hospitals, and most departments have their own written manuals relative to their particular areas. Nursing service manuals will contain policies and procedures for general or special patient care and usually cover prevention. For this reason only the points of caution are listed in the *prevention* portion of this book. The one exception is handwashing, since it is one of the most important factors in both prevention and control of disease and infection. The section on *control* contains more detailed information.

Aseptic techniques, where indicated, and general sanitary practices are the best basic measures to prevent infection and disease. The policies and procedures presented here are only suggestions that may be used as guidelines for the individual hospital in writing their infection prevention and control manual.

Handwashing

POLICY. Hands must be washed (1) between handling of individual patients (mandatory), (2) during performance of normal duties (handling dressings, urinals, bedpans, catheters, sputum, etc.), (3) after personal use of toilet, (4) after sneezing or coughing, (5) before eating, and (6) on completion of duty.

PROCEDURES (Fig. 3-1)

General procedure for normal clinical care
1. Standing well away from the sink, turn on the water and adjust it to the desired temperature.
2. Wet hands and wrists thoroughly, holding them downward over the sink to enable the water to run toward the fingertips.
3. Take a generous portion of soap from the dispenser (liquid, flake,

or powder). If bar soap is used, it must be rinsed before being returned to the dish.

4. Scrub each hand with the other, creating as much friction as possible by interlacing the fingers and moving the hands back and forth. Continue the scrubbing action for 1 or 2 minutes, until areas

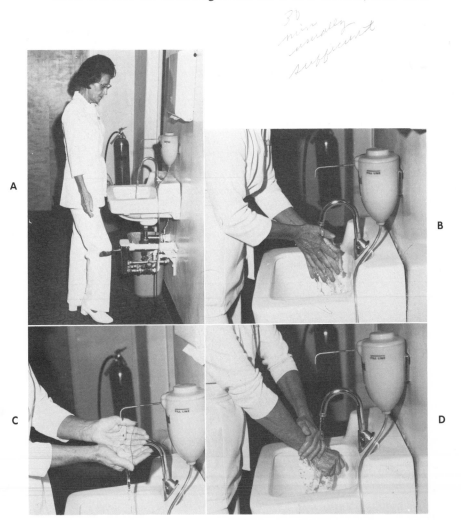

Fig. 3-1. Handwashing. **A,** Adjust water to proper temperature. **B,** Wet hands and wrists. **C,** Take a generous portion of soap. **D,** Rub hands to create friction and lather. **E,** Work nails against palms of hands. **F,** Rinse thoroughly, hands and wrists. **G,** Dry wrist and hands with paper towels. Use paper towel to turn off faucet handles.

between the fingers, the backs of hands and the palms, and areas around the fingernails are cleaned. Nails are cleaned by working them against the palms of the hands or by using an orangewood stick if necessary. ("The use of a brush is not advised because it may irritate the skin when hands are washed as often as they should in patient care."*)

5. Rinse the hands thoroughly by holding them under the running water, with elbows higher than the hands so that the water flows downward to the fingertips. All soap should be carefully removed to avoid roughened skin.

6. Dry wrists and hands with paper towels, working from the area

---

*Guide to control of infections in hospitals, Center for Disease Control, Atlanta, Georgia, p. 29.

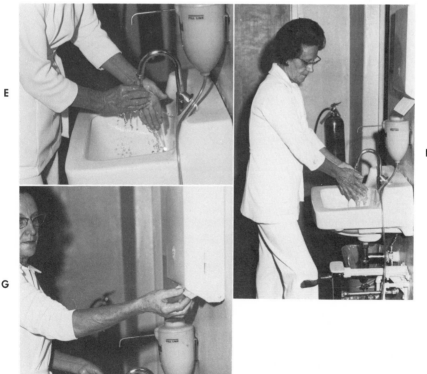

Fig. 3-1, cont'd. For legend see opposite page.

of the wrists to the fingertips. Discard each towel after one motion from wrist to fingertips.

7. Since the faucet handle is considered contaminated, turn off the water by using a dry paper towel to cover the faucet handle.

8. Apply hand lotion.

Surgical scrub. This procedure varies with the individual hospital. Personnel will don the appropriate operating room dress before beginning the scrub. Hands and arms are held *upward* so that water will drip from the elbow, and scrubbing proceeds from the fingertips toward the elbow. Water is adjusted to desired temperature and left running throughout the scrub.

1. Wet hands and arms thoroughly and apply soap.

2. Wash about one minute from the fingertips to the elbow.

3. Rinse hands and arms from fingertips to elbow.

4. Apply more soap. Using a disposable, sterile brush or sponge, scrub until the area is covered with lather (about 4 minutes).

5. Discard brush. Clean nails with a sterile orangewood stick or nail file and discard.

6. Rinse hands and arms thoroughly.

7. Apply more soap. Using a new brush or sponge, scrub hands and forearms for another 4 minutes.

8. Rinse thoroughly.

9. Use a sterile towel to blot hands and arms dry.

Personnel

POLICY. Direct or indirect patient care must be administered by personnel who are free of infection and who follow sanitary practices.

All personnel must observe the hospital's personnel health service program.

The appearance of all personnel, especially those having patient care contact, should always be neat and clean, with special emphasis on hair, uniforms, and shoes. The hair should be worn off the collar. Long hair must be contained in a net or cap.

High-risk areas:

Operating room personnel must wear scrub suits or gowns, caps, and disposable shoe covers or nonconductive shoes. Masks must be worn at all times in the operating room suite and changed frequently (always *between* cases). Masks should never be worn dangling around the neck, either in the operating area or in the hospital proper. A special hood is required for long hair, sideburns, or beards.

Nursery personnel requirements are discussed under the prevention procedure for the nursery.

Delivery and recovery room personnel must wear clean scrub gowns. These gowns should not be worn outside the service area without a cover gown.

Visitors

POLICY. Children under the age of 14 years should not be permitted to visit hospital patients.

No patient should be allowed more than two visitors at one time.

Visitors should be free of infection.

Strict controls should be exercised concerning visitors in high-risk areas.

Visitors should observe regulations concerning visiting hours.

Ventilation

POLICY

Filters and vents. Air-conditioning filters must be cleaned regularly with a bactericidal solution and disposable filters changed at regular intervals according to a priority schedule.

Prefilters and dust filters in high-risk areas should be changed every 7 to 10 days (more often if heavy dust storms occur).

The high-efficiency filter should be checked frequently and changed according to the manufacturer's directions.

Air-conditioning *vents* in high-risk areas should be cleaned bimonthly. In other hospital areas routine cleaning on a quarterly basis should be observed.

Air exchange. Adequate, frequent air exchange of 100% should be the rule in the operating room, delivery room, intensive care units, and recovery room. The recommended temperature is 68° to 70° F, and the humidity should be 50%. The rate of air exchange should be 15 to 25 air exchanges per hour.

Equipment and supplies

POLICY. Each patient's area is considered an individual unit, and on admission the patient is issued his own utensils, bedpan, urinal, washbasin, emesis basin, tissues, and other necessary items. If disposable cups and pitchers are not used, glasses should be changed daily.

Proper sterilization and decontamination of instruments *and* equipment must be maintained.

Germ-free ice must be provided.

1. Ice machines should be routinely cultured.
2. Ice scoops must be dry when not in use. (Bacteria grows and multiplies on wet surfaces.)

A disinfected *thermometer* should be used each time a temperature is taken. The use of electronic thermometers with disposable probe covers is recommended.

PROCEDURE

1. If an *ice scoop* is used, wash hands before touching the handle of the scoop.
2. After use, wipe scoop dry with a paper towel and place on a clean metal tray.
3. Once each day, the scoop and tray should be washed in a dishwasher.

Intravenous therapy

POLICY. Sterile administration of intravenous fluids and/or medications is important to the prevention of infection, especially at the insertion site. Strict asepsis must be observed at all times.

Catheter use—precautions

Use of catheters should be reserved to certain prespecified situations, including imminent or threatened cardiorespiratory arrest, the patient whose disease is uncontrollable and in whom I.V. therapy is vital, and monitoring of cardiac status in severely decompensated patients.*

1. The I.V. bottles should be checked for cracks, and the solutions inspected for cloudiness.
2. If the venipuncture is unsuccessful, the catheter must be withdrawn and a new catheter used to start the next insertion try.
3. The I.V. tubing should be changed every 24 hours and each time a new site is used.
4. Antibiotic ointment and sterile gauze 2 × 2 inches should be reapplied daily to the catheter site, preferably at the same time the tubing is changed.
5. It is recommended that the catheter site be changed every 48 hours, unless change is unadvisable due to poor veins or the critical condition of the patient. Site should be changed if the area becomes reddened, swollen, or infected with pus.
6. Thorough skin preparation with 70% alcohol or another antiseptic is essential.
7. If any purulent drainage is noted, the physician should order a culture of the area.

Hyperalimentation with special intravenous solution—precautions. If the patient requires hyperalimentation with a special intravenous solution constituted by the hospital pharmacy, a number of precautions must be observed by the attending staff.

---

*From Use of intravenous catheters, Atlanta, 1970, Center for Disease Control.

1. *Do not use* the peripheral veins for administration of this I.V. solution. Only I.V. catheters with the tip of the catheter situated in the superior vena cava or inferior vena cava should be used. Thrombosis may result if a high concentration of dextrose is given intravenously through the peripheral veins.

2. Use of aseptic technique is imperative. The composition of this I.V. solution makes it a fertile medium for bacterial growth. A minor prep is necessary to avoid infection, and the physician should wear sterile gloves.

3. All I.V. solutions used for hyperalimentation should be hung within 1 hour after being constituted. If a solution is placed in a refrigerator for later use, the pharmacy should be contacted before the infusion is begun for verification that the solution is still acceptable, and for instructions for bringing the solution to room temperature.

4. This I.V. catheter must have a special filter that will filter out most bacteria if it is properly used.

5. Tubing and filter should be changed every 24 hours. Aseptic technique must be used both when the tubing is loosened from the insertion site and when it is replaced. Do not disturb the needle site.

6. All filters, after removal, should be sent to the microbiology laboratory for culturing.

7. If cloudiness or debris in the solution, or cracks in the bottle are noted, the entire set should be removed and cultured.

Care of cardiac catheter remaining in patient—precautions. The tip of this catheter is usually placed at the junction of the superior vena cava and the right atrium.

1. Make sure that the connection between the I.V. tubing and the catheter is secure so that they do not become separated.

2. Using aseptic technique, change the dressing over the incision daily; clean the area with antiseptic; rinse with alcohol; and apply antibiotic ointment and sterile dressing.

3. Maintain the catheter with an I.V. solution as ordered by the physician, so that there is no clotting in the catheter.

4. When the catheter is ordered removed, aseptic technique must be used: cut the end of the catheter and place it in a sterile tube to be sent to the laboratory for culture and sensitivity.

Blood transfusion—precaution. The blood filter should be changed after every two units of blood if transfusion is continuous or if continuous infusion of another solution follows the blood transfusion.

Oral suction

For nursery procedure, see nursery care procedures—tracheostomy care, p. 44.

POLICY. Suction of the oropharynx with a flexible catheter is often quite ineffective. The use of the plastic disposable tonsil suction device is much more effective.

PROCEDURE
1. Wash hands thoroughly.
2. Take the catheter from the solution and flush it with normal saline solution of water. Catheter is kept in a rigid tube (a long tubelike container) that contains a tracheostomy solution consisting of 1.750 benzalkonium (aqueous Zephiran) and 0.25% acetic acid.
3. Turn on the suction machine.
4. Insert the catheter or plastic disposable tonsil suction tip gently into the back of the mouth, avoiding the roof of the mouth (to minimize gag reflex).
5. Place thumb over open end of Y tube to create suction.
6. Withdraw catheter or tonsil suction tip slowly while rotating it. If resistance is felt, remove thumb from Y tube to release suction. Suction no longer than fifteen seconds.
7. Flush catheter or tonsil suction tip thoroughly with water (from flushing bottle) after each suctioning.
8. Repeat short suctioning as necessary to keep airway open.
9. Store catheter or tonsil suction tip in tracheostomy solution. Rigid tube, catheter or tonsil suction tip, flushing bottle, and tracheostomy solution should be changed every 24 hours.

Dressings

POLICY. All soiled dressings must be bagged and placed in suitable containers—not in the patient's wastebasket.

PROCEDURE
1. Obtain dressing tray and antiseptic from designated area on the unit. Screen the patient and wash hands thoroughly.
2. Expose operative site. Use forceps to remove soiled dressings and place them in a plastic bag. The plastic bag with a *very* soiled dressing should be placed in a *paper* bag.
3. Cleanse the wound area as necessary.
4. Use sterile forceps to cover the wound with sterile dressings. Place all instruments in a wrapper to avoid contamination of the area.
5. Appearance of the wound and drainage should be noted.

Cultures

POLICY. Information on requisitions to the laboratory should include the area from which the culture is taken and the type of surgery that was performed.

PROCEDURE

1. Wash hands thoroughly. Use forceps to remove the patient's dressing. Discard dressings into a plastic bag.
2. Cleanse the skin area around the wound with suitable antiseptic solution (use forceps).
3. Using one swab at a time, obtain material for culture from the wound or from the wound drainage. (If there is no opening, there is no need to culture the skin area.)
4. Place swabs into a container immediately without contaminating swab or container. An aspirated specimen is placed in a tube with a screw-on top.
5. Wash hands and, using clean forceps, replace dressing if needed; then wash hands again.
6. Cultures must be sent immediately to the laboratory and processed within the hour.
7. Routine orders should include: smear, Gram stain, culture, and sensitivities for pathogens.
8. Sensitivities should always be done on positive cultures obtained from blood, urine, all operating room specimens, and specimens obtained from body cavities.

Urinary system

POLICY. A closed drainage system should be used for each patient who has an indwelling (Foley) catheter. The closed system prevents entry of bacteria into the body.

PROCEDURE

Drainage system

1. Hang the drainage bag straight on the bed frame. Do not let it touch the floor.
2. Keep the filter dry and the end of the drain covered (to prevent bacteria from entering the bag).

Catheter care (male or female patient)

1. Wash meatus thoroughly and rinse well.
2. Cleanse the catheter of all dried blood and secretions. Wash the general perineal area and legs to avoid irritation and discomfort to the patient.
3. Apply ointment with sterile applicator to meatus if ordered by the physician.
4. Check the patient's rectal area, and wash, if necessary, to help prevent fecal contamination of the catheter.

Clean voided urine specimens. Ambulatory patients may obtain their own specimen if properly instructed; otherwise the procedure is performed by nursing personnel.

1. To obtain a clean voided urine specimen from a male patient:
   a. Cleanse the penis thoroughly with an antiseptic towelette (soap may retard growth in the specimen if not rinsed off with sterile water). Pay special attention to the area under the foreskin.
   b. Ask the patient to void a small amount into the urinal. This portion eliminates surface contamination and is discarded.
   c. Ask the patient to then void into a sterile container. Cap the container and send it to the laboratory. (A second bottle may be used to collect a portion of the urine for culture and sensitivity, if ordered.)
2. To obtain a clean voided urine specimen from a female patient:
   a. Cleanse external genitalia, using a towelette and wiping the perineum backward toward the anus.
   b. Separate the labia and cleanse with a second wipe. Discard wipe.
   c. Place a cotton ball in the vagina to prevent contamination from vaginal secretions.
   d. Holding the labia apart, ask the patient to void a small amount into the bedpan, to eliminate surface contamination.
   e. Collect the specimen midstream, into a sterile collection container. Cap the container and send it to the laboratory.

Linen

POLICY. Bed linen should be changed (at least) daily.

Mattresses, pillow covers, and blankets should be washed and disinfected before being used by another patient.

The linen on tables or carts used for patient diagnosis or treatment should be changed after each use. Wheelchairs or carts not covered with linen, if not visibly soiled, should be sprayed with a disinfectant before using.

PROCEDURE

Soiled linen. This method contains the germs inside the bag so that they cannot become airborne throughout the hospital when soiled linen is moved from the unit to the laundry.

1. Use thick cloth bags (such as ticking) for the individual patient's soiled linen each time linen is removed from the bed or patient. (Do not use pillowcases.)
2. Leave room at the top of the bag so that the bag may be folded over for convenience in carrying it to the soiled linen area.
3. Never throw the linen on the patient's floor or on top of the hamper

in the soiled linen area. It should be placed in the linen hamper without being removed from the individual laundry bag.

Handling clean linen in the laundry

1. All laundry personnel must wear clean uniforms.
2. Hands must be washed after handling any soiled supplies.
3. Linen must be kept from clothing contact with attendants.
4. Clean linen must never be stored on the floor, even if it is in bags.
5. All linen closets must be kept closed when not in use.
6. Linen shelves must be cleaned frequently.
7. Monthly cultures should be taken in the laundry area.

Miscellaneous prevention policies and procedures

POLICY. Special areas, such as operating rooms and delivery rooms, should be routinely cultured.

Eye drops with a one-unit dosage and nasal sprays should be dispensed as prescribed.

Each surgical patient should be instructed in, and should practice, preoperative and postoperative deep breathing and coughing, to prevent pneumonia.

Cleaning

POLICY. All patient areas should be cleaned daily, including the exterior of equipment. There should be terminal cleaning of rooms or patient areas after each patient's discharge and before another patient is admitted. Floors, faucets, washbasins, and exposed supplies throughout the hospital are considered contaminated.

The *environmental services* department is responsible for sanitation—routinely keeping the hospital sanitarily clean and aesthetically acceptable.

Cleaning procedures must be established to create a safe, bacteria-controlled environment. Floors are the most highly contaminated areas, and if they are not properly cleaned, shoes and wheels will pick up germs from the floors and spread them from room to room.

Preventing odors is better than controlling them later, and cleaning creates a more pleasant atmosphere. Cleaning requirements differ with hospitals, and methods change frequently. For up-to-date information, contact the Center for Disease Control, Atlanta, Georgia.

PROCEDURE

General cleaning after discharge. The purpose of this procedure is to provide a safe, attractive environment for the patient. Cleaning equipment, a good germicide, and clean utensils should be assembled and taken into the room.

1. Strip bed completely and place soiled linen, including the plastic mattress cover, in the laundry bag.
2. Dispose of excess equipment that has been left by the discharged patient, and remove all utensils that are not disposable to the "dirty" utility room, to be cleaned.
3. Be sure to use the correct dilution of cleaning solution. If it is too strong, it may cause dermatitis; if too weak, it will be ineffective.
4. Spray and wash the bedside chair. Spray the pillow and place it on the clean chair. Spray the rubber drawsheet on both sides.
5. Spray the mattress on both sides until damp. Pay particular attention to seams and buttons, since germs and dust collect in crevices.
6. Fold the mattress from its end toward the center and wash the exposed bed frame and springs. Repeat the procedure, working from the opposite end.
7. Change the cleaning solution when necessary.
8. Damp-dust shelves and inside of closet, lights, air-conditioning unit, signal light, doors, and windows and sills; spot-wash the walls.
9. Spray and wash all furniture and fixtures of the unit (bedside table, overbed table, bedside lamp, cupboards).
10. Clean bathroom and replenish supplies as necessary.
    a. Flush toilet, and clean both sides of the toilet seat, fixtures, metal hinges, pipes, and collars with a cloth that has been dampened in disinfectant detergent solution.
    b. Clean the outside of the toilet bowl. Use a brush if it is heavily soiled. Dry with a cloth.
    c. Scrub the inside of the toilet bowl with the toilet brush and and abrasive cleaner, paying special attention to the rim and trap.
    d. Rinse well and flush.
    e. Clean the sink with abrasive cleanser and disinfectant detergent solution. Tub and shower should be flushed with an alkaline solution after cleaning, and then dried.
11. Remove cleaning supplies from the room; make the bed with clean linen; place utensils in proper place and add fresh supply of disposable items in the cupboard.
12. Mop the floor with clean germicidal solution.
13. Leave the furniture in straight alignment and make a last-minute inspection of the unit and bathroom to be sure it is ready for occupancy.
14. Report any breakage or repairs needed to the immediate supervisor.

Cleaning x-ray department

1. Clean all control boards, panels, lights, and sensitive equipment with disposable cloth soaked in alcohol. Alcohol is quickly evaporated, thereby providing a safety factor.
2. Keep all ventilators clean and free of dirt and grime; vacuum the fan outlet parts on x-ray equipment once each week.
3. Clean and mop the floors each night with germicide solution.
4. Portable x-ray equipment
   a. Wash with alcohol each night.
   b. Before replacing portable units in storage rooms, clean the storage room shelves and floor, and spot-wash the walls with germicide detergent solution.

Cleaning operating room between all cases

1. Remove linen from operating table, pillow, and arm board and discard in laundry hamper.
2. Empty wastebaskets and replace plastic liners.
3. Remove filled laundry bag from hamper, wipe hamper with germicide solution, and place a clean laundry bag in the hamper.
4. Scrub floor with germicide solution, and follow with wet vacuum technique.
5. Wipe table, stand, buckets, I.V. poles, and stools with germicide solution.
6. Make up table with clean linen.
7. Empty and rinse suction bottles. Replace clean tubing as needed. Return wrapped sterile supplies and suture boxes to the proper place.
8. Replace all items in proper places.

Nursery care
PROCEDURES
Personnel

1. Wear hair neatly groomed, not touching the collar, and contained in a hairnet at all times.
2. Before entering the nursery area, change to a fresh scrub gown. Uniforms or street clothing should not be worn into the nursery area.
3. Do not wear rings or a watch in the nursery area (a plain wedding band is usually an exception). A watch may be pinned to the pocket of the scrub gown.
4. Do not use fingernail polish. Keep nails clean and neat.
5. Do not work in the nursery area if any of the following is present:
   a. Symptoms of diarrhea or upper respiratory infection.
   b. Cold sores or fever blisters.

      c. Any lesion on the genitals or irritating vaginal discharge.

      d. Skin infection or pustular acne.

  6. Nursing personnel will have a chest x-ray examination every twelve months.

  7. Do not take magazines or food into the work areas of the nursery.

  8. Personnel who work in either a regular or a special nursery are not to return to the nursery within the same 8-hour shift after having worked in another area of the hospital. They are not to work in isolation areas (except nursery isolation).

  9. Wash well with bacteriostatic soap for three minutes, from fingertips to elbows, before starting to work in the nursery. Hands must be rewashed if face is inadvertently touched.

10. Wash hands with bacteriostatic soap between handling of each baby.

11. Change to a uniform on leaving the nursery department; on returning to the nursery, change into a clean scrub gown. Scrub gowns worn outside the area must be changed before the area is entered again. A clean cover gown may be worn over the scrub gown and removed when personnel return to the nursery.

12. Do not hold a baby next to face or hair:

      a. Never kiss a baby.

      b. When burping a baby, hold him over the shoulder on a clean diaper.

13. All physicians and other personnel entering the ICU nursery should wash their hands and put on a clean gown.

14. All physicians and other personnel entering the *regular* nursery should wash their hands. Gowns need not be worn if neither equipment nor baby is handled.

Signs of infection

The responsible physician or his alternate should be notified at once in the event of any of the following:

  1. Any serious change in the infant's condition

  2. Signs of infection

      a. Diarrhea

      b. Blood in stools

      c. Inflammed umbilicus

      d. Suspicious skin lesion (questionable lesions should be cultured)

      e. Eye discharge

  3. Marked change in respiration—apnea or cyanosis

Feeding

  1. Preparation of mother's room

a. Turn bedspread down halfway.
b. Draw curtains.
c. Turn the light on over the bed (during night shift).
d. Leave room door open.
e. Lay infant on top sheet—never in bed with the mother.
2. Preparation of mother
   a. Pull nightgown down from shoulder—NEVER up from soiled areas. If it cannot be pulled down or unbuttoned, it must be removed completely and replaced with a hospital gown.
   b. Wash breasts (nipple area) with soap-and-water sponges.
   c. Wash hands with soap and water.
   d. Nonnursing mothers need only wash hands.

Preparation for physician's examination

1. Wash hands with bacteriostatic soap and water.
2. Remove infant's shirt.
3. Unpin diaper, change diaper if it is soiled, and close safety pins.
4. Take bassinet to the work area when the physician arrives.
5. Tell the physician the baby's weight.
6. Clean stethoscope bell with an alcohol sponge.
7. Assist the physician with the entire examination.
8. When the examination is completed, dress the baby and return it with the bassinet to the proper nursery.
9. Wash hands.

Daily routine for intensive care

1. Babies in intensive care are never taken to examining rooms.
2. Incubators should be changed every 7 days.
3. Nurses who work in the intensive care unit must be particularly conscious of handwashing technique and personal care of self. High-risk infants are very susceptible to infection.
4. A cover gown will be worn by every person leaving the special nursery for any reason and removed when personnel return to the nursery.
5. Parents of an infant in the special nursery must wash and gown to enter the nursery either to visit, touch, or hold the infant, as determined by the physician. The number of visits and the length of each visit should be determined by the charge nurse. In case of an emergency, all viewing and visits are curtailed.

Intramuscular injections

All injections are to be administered only on order of the physician.
1. Wash hands with bacteriostatic soap and water.

2. Prepare required amount of medication. A No. 25 needle is recommended for all injections except penicillin (a No. 23 needle is used).
3. Cleanse area of injection with an alcohol sponge.
4. Chart medication, amount and site of injection, and the time administered.

Isolette cleaning procedures

Isolette is cleaned every 4 days if moisture is used; otherwise, it is cleaned every 7 days.

1. Assemble needed equipment at the sink area.
2. Mix disinfectant solution in a basin. Empty water reservoir. Take the port rings and front opening gasket off and place them in a cleaning sink. Remove the plug. Remove the power pack and wash it.
3. Wash the entire surface of the Isolette, inside and out, with cleaning solution and dry it with a clean cloth.
4. Place fresh cleaning solution in the reservoir during the cleaning process. After all of the surface is washed, use a small brush in the opening from inside and through the full pipe from the outside. Drain and rinse with 0.25% acetic acid and then rinse with distilled water. Wipe dry with clean cloth.
5. Wash the power pack thoroughly with cleaning solution. Clean the wheels with applicators soaked in disinfectant solution. If film remains, alcohol may be used. Twill tape or pipe cleaners, saturated with cleaning solution, may be eased under the wheel to catch the lint.
6. Reassemble the unit, plug it in, and set the temperature.

Tracheostomy care

1. Suctioning of tube requires the following procedures:
   a. Wash hands thoroughly and put on sterile gloves.
   b. Attach sterile disposable catheter to suction apparatus and turn on the machine.
   c. Insert catheter gently through tube openings (at least 2 inches).
   d. Place thumb over opening in tube.
   e. Withdraw catheter slowly while rotating it.
   f. Suction no longer than 15 seconds.
   g. Flush catheter thoroughly with solution after each suctioning.
   h. Repeat suctioning as necessary to keep airway open.
   i. Discard suction catheter.
2. Recommendations for care of suction and mist equipment are as follows:

a. Use only sterile distilled water.

b. Suction equipment should be disposable plastic and changed and discarded every day.

c. Nurses are instructed that the suction bottle is to be treated as a contaminated area. Careful handwashing is mandatory after handling.

d. A fresh, sterilized suction bottle is used daily.

Control (isolation) policies and procedures

Infection control procedures are constantly being modified to keep up-to-date with new developments. There will always be conflicting evidence as to the effectiveness of specific control policies and procedures. Thus there will be a wide variance among hospitals. The policies and procedures listed here have been successfully used and may be easily adapted to the individual hospital's requirements. Repetition of some policies, procedures, and categories is unavoidable.

Admission of patient to isolation

POLICY

Admission order. A physician's written order must be obtained before a patient is admitted or discharged from isolation. The physician is also responsible for reporting all diseases to the state health department.

Room (Fig. 3-2). Private rooms are to be used when indicated, especially for isolation in the reverse and strict categories. Multiple rooms may be used for patients with the same disease, if the attending physicians agree.

In pediatrics, under controlled conditions, patients with certain respiratory diseases such as croup and pneumonia may be placed in a ward setting. Private rooms should be available when stricter techniques are indicated, as with plague and smallpox.

All surfaces within a patient's room are considered contaminated, including walls, floors, windows, doorknobs, and bathroom.

PROCEDURE

Preparation of room for isolation. This procedure is applicable to strict isolation but may be modified for any category.

1. Remove from the room all unnecessary supplies that cannot be washed.

2. Supply the bedside stand with utensils, tissues, disposable pitcher and cups, lotion, and bedside paper bags.

3. As a convenience to the patient, pin a paper bag to the bed for disposal of soiled tissues.

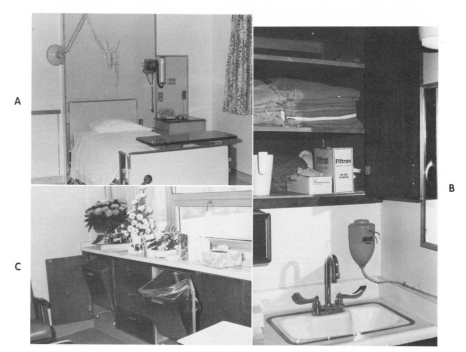

Fig. 3-2. Isolation rooms. **A,** Private room with or without anteroom. **B,** Anteroom with supply cupboard and sink. **C,** Private room with anteroom having linen and waste bins opening to outside of building for removal of waste and linen.

4. Place towels and bactericidal soap in the bathroom.
5. Line the linen hamper and wastebasket with plastic liners and place the hamper near the door.
6. Place an isolation cart convenient to the room.

The isolation cart (Fig. 3-3) may be a utility table on wheels or a specially designed cart. A pullout front shelf and a stationary side shelf of the cart may be used for a work area, or for placement of diet, medicine, or laboratory trays. A hook on the side of the cart may be used for the physician's or visitor's coat. A rack on the side of the cart may hold a box of masks, and brochures explaining isolation procedures. The cart is stocked with paper and plastic bags, gowns, gloves, linen, red laundry bags, category door cards, and a roll of isolation tape for marking contaminated items. The cart should be cleaned daily by the floor personnel and restocked for each shift. When the cart is no longer needed, it should be cleaned, restocked, and returned to a storage area for future use. It is

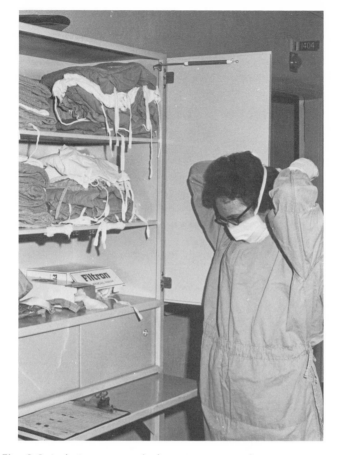

Fig. 3-3. Isolation cart used when private room has no anteroom.

never taken inside the contaminated room. It is a convenient backup for personnel who care for the isolated patient.

Admission of patient. This procedure is used for very strict isolation. However, it may be modified for use with less virulent diseases.

The patient should be admitted directly to the isolation room to avoid contact with other patients, visitors, or personnel. If the nurse epidemiologist is not already aware of the admission, she should be promptly notified.

A door card identifying the precautions and the category of isolation is placed on the door. All requisition slips to other departments for their services to the patient should be marked "Isolation," and the category of isolation (for example, enteric or strict) should be noted.

The nurse should remove watch and rings before entering the isolation room. The watch may be taken into the room on a clean paper towel, which is placed on another paper towel in the contaminated area.

The patient and his family should be helped to understand their responsibility in carrying out correct isolation techniques. Clothing of the patient should be wrapped in a clean, uncontaminated bag and sent home with the family, where they should be aired or exposed to sunlight for 24 hours, and then washed, dry-cleaned, or disinfected. If the family is not present, the clothes should be kept in a plastic bag in the room with the patient. It is important that both the patient and his family be instructed in the proper use of tissues to cover his mouth when coughing, and in the disposal of the tissue after use.

Articles that cannot be disinfected or autoclaved, or that are not disposable, should remain outside the room whenever possible. Disposable items should be used if available.

1. Wash hands, don mask and gown if indicated, and assist the patient in the removal of his clothing. Place the patient's clothing and personal effects in a plastic bag and instruct the family in protective measures.
2. An assistant outside the room holds a clean plastic bag while the nurse inside the room places the contaminated bag of clothing and personal effects into it, taking care not to contaminate the outside of the clean bag. The bag is left outside the room for the family to take with them when they leave.
3. Take the patient's temperature, pulse, and respiration and collect a urine specimen.
4. Place an identification bracelet on his wrist and a small piece of tape, color-coded to the category of isolation and the door card, on the wristband. Another strip of the colored tape is placed on the patient's chart cover, along with an isolation label.
5. Instruct the patient in hospital routine and make him comfortable. Answer all his questions as thoroughly as possible, and check to make sure that all necessary items are convenient to him.
6. Wash hands and remove the mask and then the gown. Place the mask in the wastebasket and the gown in the linen hamper.
7. Wash hands again before leaving the room.

Patient's chart and requisitions

POLICY. The patient's chart should not be taken into the patient's room. It should be left on the shelf of an isolation cart or at the nurses' station.

Requisitions to other departments, such as x-ray and laboratory, must be labeled with the category of isolation.

When the patient is scheduled for surgery, the operating room must be notified that the patient is in isolation and the category of care that is being used.

Handwashing

POLICY. Hands must be washed before entering or leaving isolation rooms. Strict handwashing is mandatory before and after patient care.

PROCEDURE

Use procedure for handwashing that is detailed in the prevention portion of this chapter, with two exceptions: do not use bar soap, and wash and rinse the hands twice instead of once.

Masks

POLICY. Masks are worn to prevent the spread of air-borne infectious droplets. The mask may be worn by either patient or nurse. When gown or gloves are worn, the mask is adjusted first. Strings of the mask are considered clean.

Masks should be changed frequently, since the moisture that gathers promotes the growth of bacteria.

PROCEDURE (Fig. 3-4)

1. Wash hands and pick up mask by the strings. Adjust mask snugly over the nose and mouth.
2. Tie the top strings first to about ear level.
3. Do not touch the front of the mask while it is being worn, since the front is considered contaminated.
4. To remove the mask, wash hands and untie top and bottom strings. Hold the mask by the strings and drop it into the wastebasket.

Gowns

POLICY. A gown is worn to protect visitors or personnel from direct-contact contamination with the patient's secretions and excretions or his surroundings. It should be long enough to completely cover the uniform, and must never be worn outside the isolation area.

Neckbands, ties, and inside of the gown are considered clean.

In *pediatrics,* nursing personnel will wear green scrub gowns. If a ward clerk must assist a patient in isolation, the clerk should put on a clean isolation gown, tie it properly, and remove the gown when duties with the patient are completed. Hands should always be washed.

In *pediatrics,* if it is necessary to care for "clean" patients after caring for isolation patients, the attendant should change back to a uniform or into a clean scrub gown.

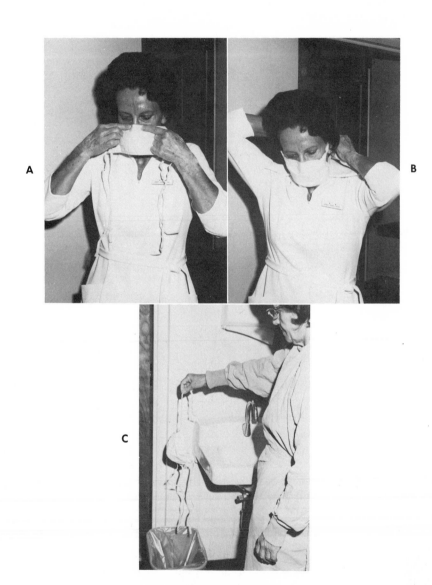

Fig. 3-4. Masking. **A,** Adjust mask to nose. **B,** Tie strings in comfortable position. **C,** Discard mask in patient's wastebasket after use. Always hold mask by the strings.

PROCEDURE (Figs. 3-5 and 3-6)

1. Before donning gown, wash hands. Slip hands between the back hems of the gown and shoulders. Hold arms high, allowing sleeves to fall over arms. Tie neck strings.
2. For maximum coverage, hold edges of back hems with each hand and overlap the gown in the back. Tie waist strings securely.
3. To remove gown, unfasten waist ties.
4. Wash hands and unfasten neck ties.
5. Slip one hand under the cuff of the opposite sleeve and pull the sleeve over the hand.
6. Grasp the opposite sleeve with the hand that is covered by the sleeve, and pull the sleeve over the hand.
7. Fold the contaminated side of the gown, which contains bacteria, inside and roll the gown.
8. Discard the gown in the linen hamper.
9. Wash hands.

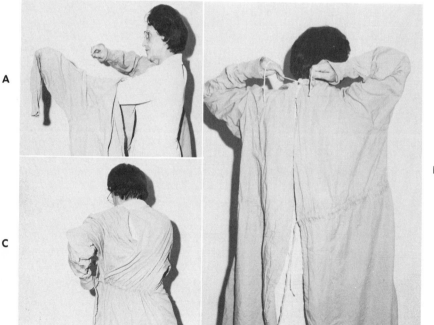

Fig. 3-5. Gowning. **A,** Slip hands between hems of gown and shoulders. **B,** Tie neck strings. **C,** Overlap gown in back and tie waist strings.

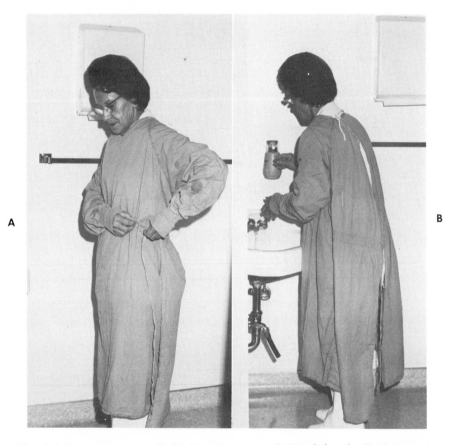

Fig. 3-6. Removing gown. **A,** Untie waist strings. **B,** Wash hands. **C,** Untie neck strings. **D,** Slip hands out of gown, preventing uniform contamination. **E,** Fold inside of gown over outside. **F,** Roll in a ball and discard in the linen hamper.

Gloves

POLICY. Gloves must be worn when indicated.

Sterile gloves are used to prevent cross contamination or increased infection when changing dressings.

Nonsterile gloves are used to protect hands against contamination by feces, urine of patients with enteric diseases.

Gloves do not replace handwashing.

PROCEDURE (Fig. 3-7)

1. Gloves are put on after the gown in order that the glove cuffs may be drawn up over the gown sleeves.

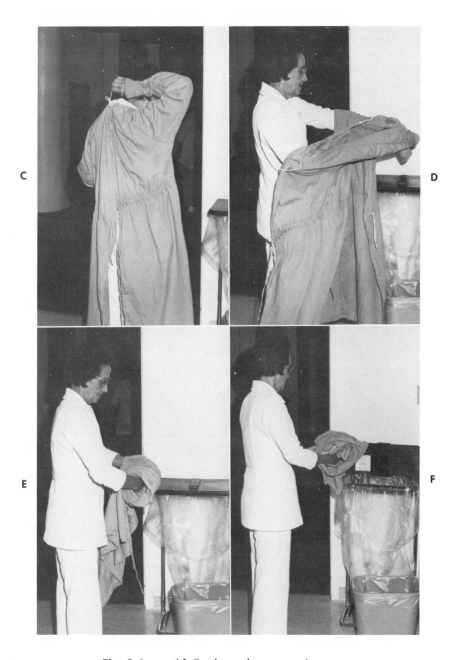

Fig. 3-6, cont'd. For legend see opposite page.

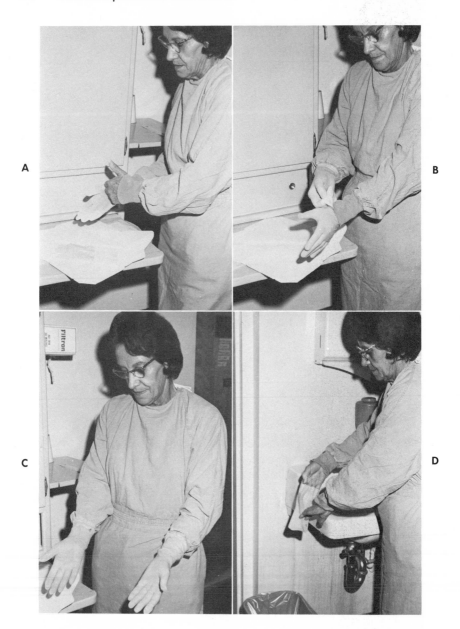

Fig. 3-7. Gloving. **A,** Insert hand under cuff of right glove and pull glove into place. **B,** Insert gloved hand under left cuff and pull glove into place. **C,** Cover gown wrists with glove cuffs. **D,** Discard glove into patient's waste container after use.

2. Most sterile gloves are packaged with a 2-inch cuff. Grasp the inside of the cuff of the right glove with the left hand. Insert the right hand and pull the glove into place.
3. The gloved hand is inserted under the cuff of the left glove. Insert the left hand in the left glove and pull it into place. Pull the glove cuff over the wrist of the gown.
4. Gloves should be removed before mask or gown, and discarded in the wastebasket.
5. Hands should be washed after gloves are removed.

Visitors

POLICY. Although instructing and preparing visitors for isolation visitation is time-consuming and often frustrating to the nursing staff, their presence is valuable to the emotional well-being of the patient. Many hospitals limit visitors to one and the length of stay to 20 minutes. However, this is a judgment the individual hospital must make.

No more than two visitors at any one time should be allowed, and the length of stay should be governed by the needs of the patient.

PROCEDURE

1. Before *entering* the room, visitors must inquire at the nurses station for instructions, and for gowns and masks if indicated.
2. Visitors' hats and coats should be left outside the room. Only articles that can be discarded, disinfected, or sterilized should be taken into the room.
3. It is recommended that purses be left with relatives outside the room. However, if a visitor must carry a purse or other articles into the room, the articles must be placed in a clean paper bag. The bag must not be opened in the room until just before leaving.
4. Before *leaving* the room, the visitors must wash hands, and then remove mask and gown. Discard mask in wastebasket and gown in linen hamper. Wash hands again.
5. If articles have been taken into the room, follow this procedure:
   a. Before removing the gown, open the paper bag containing the articles, opening it wide enough to remove the articles without touching the bag again.
   b. Do not remove articles at this time.
   c. Wash hands.
   d. Place a clean paper towel on the floor. Remove articles and place them on the clean paper towel.
   e. Place contaminated paper bag in the wastebasket.
   f. Remove mask and gown. Discard mask in wastebasket and gown in linen hamper.

g. Wash hands again.

h. Use a clean paper towel to open the door, and discard the towel in the wastebasket.

i. Carefully take the articles from the paper towel and carry them from the room. The paper towel on the floor may be discarded later by nursing personnel.

Personnel

POLICY. An employee exposed to an undiagnosed infectious disease must notify his department supervisor so that correct protective measures can be instituted (for example, gamma globulin for hepatitis, and x-ray examination and skin testing for active tuberculosis).

All personnel from other departments who enter an isolation unit must follow all precautions and procedures provided for that area.

Personnel who have cared for isolation patients on any one day in pediatrics should not "float" to a clean ward.

If a patient is admitted and subsequently diagnosed as having measles, the physicians of all other patients that were exposed must be notified. This is usually the responsibility of the nurse in charge of the ward.

In the *pediatric* area, it is usually the nurse who must take the precautions.

Taking temperature, pulse, and respiration (TPR)

POLICY. The most aseptic method for taking temperatures is to use a clean thermometer each time a temperature is taken. For other procedures, consult publications from the Center for Disease Control.

PROCEDURE

1. Leave pencil and paper on the isolation cart shelf outside the room.
2. Don gown and mask as indicated.
3. Bring clean thermometer and a paper towel into the room.
4. Place the paper towel on the overbed table and place wristwatch on the towel.
5. Remove thermometer from packet. Lay packet on a clean towel next to watch.
6. Follow usual TPR procedure.
7. Place the thermometer (after wiping it with an alcohol sponge) soiled tip down in the packet. Do not touch outside of the packet.
8. Wash hands, remove gown, and wash hands again.
9. Pick up watch and packet; discard paper towel in the wastebasket, taking care to touch only the clean surface of the paper towel.
10. Place the packet in a paper bag and set the bag, open side up, on a shelf of the cart until the end of the shift.

11. Record TPR after leaving the room and transfer notation to clinical record. See step 1.
12. At the end of each shift, seal thermometers in a bag. Mark the bag "Isolation thermometers" and place in pick-up area for sterilization.
13. If disposable thermometers are used, leave in patient's room until discharge. Disinfect before use by wiping with alcohol sponge. After discharge, destroy thermometer. Do not send home with patient.

Taking blood pressure

POLICY. The sphygmomanometer and stethoscope are to be kept in the room for the duration of isolation.

PROCEDURE
1. *If blood pressure apparatus is used for only one patient,* observe the following procedure:
   a. Leave paper and pencil on the shelf of the isolation cart outside the room.
   b. Don gown and mask if indicated.
   c. Wipe stethoscope with alcohol sponges before use.
   d. Follow the usual procedure for taking blood pressure.
   e. Wash hands.
   f. Remove gown and discard in hamper.
   g. Repeat handwashing.
   h. Chart blood pressure reading after leaving the room. See step 1a.
2. *If blood pressure apparatus must be used for other patients,* observe the following procedure:
   a. Have patient wear a clean, long-sleeved gown.
   b. Place cuff over the clean sleeve of gown.
   c. When blood pressure apparatus is removed from the sleeve, place it on a clean paper towel.
   d. Wash hands.
   e. Remove blood pressure apparatus from paper towel. Spray with disinfectant all the surfaces that have touched the patient. *Do not use for 20 minutes.*
   f. Wash hands.

Dietary service

POLICY. Dietary service should be notified immediately both when a patient is placed in isolation and when he is removed from isolation.

All dietary service utensils used in isolation are usually disposable.

If the patient requests regular silverware, it is to be washed after each meal, folded in a paper towel, and left in the patient's room. After the patient is discharged, it is sent to central service for steam sterilization before being returned to dietary service.

Nursing personnel are responsible for serving and picking up food trays. Dietary service personnel, except for dietitians, are not permitted to enter the patient's room.

All disposable trays, food, and disposable utensils are disposed of by double bagging.

PROCEDURE
1. Wash hands before picking up tray.
2. Don gown and mask if indicated.
3. Take tray with disposable dishes into the patient's room and place on overbed table.
4. Make the patient comfortable and provide a good eating position. If patient is on bed rest, offer patient a wet washcloth and dry towel so that he can wash his hands.
5. If the patient can feed himself, wash hands, remove and discard gown, rewash hands, and leave the room.
6. If the patient must be fed, take time to make the experience enjoyable.
7. When the patient has finished eating:
   a. Discard leftover liquids in toilet or down sink drain.
   b. Place solids and disposable dishes in a plastic bag. Tie or seal the bag and discard it in the wastebasket.
8. Wash hands, remove gown, repeat handwashing, and leave the room.

Dressings

POLICY. Dressings from isolation patients are to be placed in a double plastic bag, tied securely at the top, and placed in the appropriate container. (Container must have a lid and plastic liner. It may be marked with a bright color, an indication that it is to be used only for surgical dressings.)

PROCEDURE
1. Place dressings in a plastic or paper bag and discard in the proper container.
2. Dressings should not be placed in any other container on the patient's unit, nor should they be disposed of in the city disposal system.
3. The plastic bag containing the dressings should be removed daily from the container and incinerated.

Isolation waste

POLICY. All isolation wastes should be incinerated.

All waste must be double bagged and marked "Isolation."
Needles and glass syringes should not be put into wastebaskets.

PROCEDURE
Wastebaskets

1. Don gown and mask if indicated.
2. Remove the plastic bag from the wastebasket by grasping the top edges.
3. Tie the top of the plastic bag with a knot or seal with tape.
4. Follow procedure for double bagging of contaminated supplies.
5. Discard the double bag, clearly marked "Isolation" in the proper container.

Body wastes

1. Nasopharyngeal secretions and sputum
   a. Instruct the patient to cover mouth and nose when sneezing or coughing, and to expectorate into tissues.
   b. Tissues are discarded into the bag pinned to the bedside—not directly into the wastebasket.
   c. When bedside bags are partially filled, seal the top with tape and drop into patient's wastebasket.
   d. Wash hands.
2. Feces, urine, vomitus, liquids, and foods
   a. Don gown and mask if indicated.
   b. Discard excreta or liquid into toilet and flush. Be careful not to splash.
   c. Wash and rinse container well and replace in proper location.
   d. Wash hands.

Linen

POLICY. All contaminated linen must be double bagged. The outside bag is red, designating contaminated linen.

PROCEDURE
Double bagging of linen (Fig. 3-8). A hamper frame with a plastic liner on the frame is placed inside the room near the door. When the bag is two-thirds full of soiled linen it should be double bagged before being placed in the soiled linen room. The double-bagging procedure requires the aid of an assistant who remains outside the isolation room to prevent contamination of the outside bag.

1. Inside the room: Don gown and mask if indicated, and remove the plastic liner, which is filled with soiled linen, from the hamper frame. Close the top of the liner with a wire closure and carry the bag to the doorway.

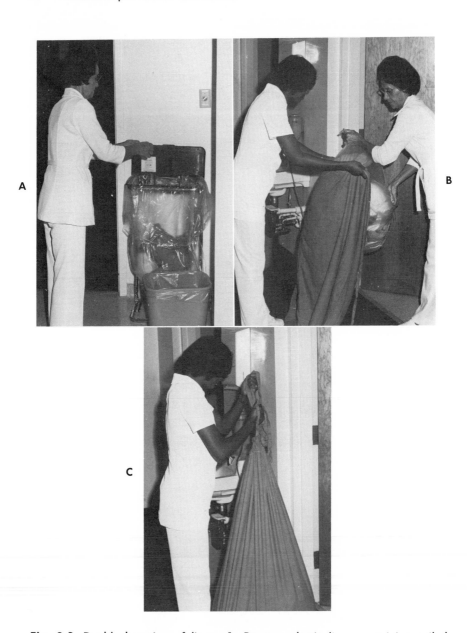

Fig. 3-8. Double bagging of linen. **A,** Remove plastic liner containing soiled linen, close top of liner, and take bag to doorway. **B,** Assistant outside door cuffs the red isolation bag over hands. The plastic bag is then placed in the red isolation bag. **C,** Assistant closes red bag and takes it to the linen pickup area.

2. Outside the door: The assistant cuffs a clean red laundry bag over her hands. Nurse, from inside the doorway, places the contaminated bag inside the red laundry bag. Assistant closes the red bag and secures it. Outside of bag must remain uncontaminated at all times.
3. Red bag is placed in soiled-linen area.
4. Nurse places a clean plastic liner on the hamper frame inside the room and washes hands.

Handling contaminated linen in the laundry

1. Laundry pick-up personnel: take double-bagged, contaminated laundry bag to the laundry isolation storage area.
2. Laundry attendant
   a. Don mask and gown.
   b. Open red bag and the plastic liner. Holding the bottom of the bag, dump contents of the bag into the washer.
   c. Red bags are placed in the washer; liners are washed in a separate washer used for plastic. If water-soluble bags are used, the red bag need not be opened.
   d. Wash hands.
   e. Remove mask and gown after all isolation linen has been placed into the washers, and place the gown into the washer. Masks are disposed of in the wastebasket.

Medications
PROCEDURE
Oral medication

1. Leaving medex and tray outside the room, pour medication according to hospital routine. Take medication in a paper cup on a tray to the shelf outside the patient's room.
2. Don mask and gown if indicated. (Use of gown may be eliminated if patient is cooperative.)
3. Take medication into the room.
4. Administer according to hospital procedure and discard medicine cup in the wastebasket.
5. Wash hands.
6. Remove gown.
7. Wash hands.
8. Chart medications on medex after leaving room.

Injection (subcutaneous and intramuscular)

1. Prepare medication according to hospital routine.
2. Take medication on tray to shelf outside unit and leave both tray and medex outside the room.

3. Don mask and gown if indicated.
4. Take syringe into the room and give injection according to hospital procedure.
5. Reapply needle protector and bend needle.
6. Place needle and syringe on paper towel. (They are deposited in an isolation box for needles and syringes at the nurses station, on leaving the room.) Do not leave in patient's room.
7. Wash hands and remove gown and discard.
8. Repeat handwashing.
9. Chart medications on medex on leaving the room.

Intravenous infusion (I.V. fluids)

1. The intake and output sheet is left outside the room.
2. Before entering the room, label and time-tape the I.V. bottle.
3. Wash hands.
4. The person starting the infusion will don gown, and mask if indicated.
5. Follow procedure for starting I.V. fluids.
6. Wash hands and remove gown, and rewash hands.
7. *After completion of I.V. therapy,* spray bottles and tubing with disinfectant and place the empty I.V. bottles in a paper bag. Keep the outside of the bag clean and place the bag on a clean paper towel. Seal the bag and discard in regular refuse.
8. Tubing or dressings are placed in a paper bag and discarded in the wastebasket.
9. Spray bent needles with disinfectant and carry them on a paper towel to the nurses station for disposal in the isolation needle-and-syringe box.
10. Wash hands.

Handling money from isolation patient

POLICY. Money collected from an isolation area should first be sprayed with a disinfectant. (This policy is not mandatory; it is used only to alleviate apprehension of personnel.)

PROCEDURE

1. Place coins on two paper towels.
2. Spray coins well with disinfectant. Wait a few minutes and place the sprayed coins with other money.
3. Discard paper towels in wastebasket and wash hands.

Signing of documents

PROCEDURE

1. Wash hands and don gown and mask if indicated.

2. Place two open paper towels on the patient's overbed table.
3. Place the document on the paper towels.
4. Ask the patient to read the document without handling it. If the patient must handle the document, have him wash his hands thoroughly. If the patient is in respiratory isolation, he must wear a mask.
5. Cover the document with two paper towels, leaving exposed space for the signature. The patient should use his own pen. If another pen is used and his hands have not been washed, spray the pen with disinfectant.
6. After signing, slide the document out without contaminating either hands or document.
7. Place the document on clean paper outside the door.
8. Discard paper towels, and gown if worn, and wash hands.

Outgoing mail
PROCEDURE

1. The patient should wash his hands before writing.
2. If the patient is on respiratory isolation, especially if he is coughing or expectorating profusely, a mask should be worn when writing letters.
3. Seal and stamp the envelopes at the nurses station.
4. Letters are not sterilized except in cases of smallpox.

Collection of specimens
POLICY

Patient's room. All isolation specimens must be clearly marked and placed in a marked paper bag. The outside of the container is considered clean. The bag acts as an extra protection in the event of spillage, and it is also used by the laboratory to hold contaminated tapes while the specimen is being processed.

Laboratory. All specimens from an isolation unit are to be completely enclosed within a paper bag. The outside of the bag should remain clean and should be clearly marked "Isolation."

All labels and requisitions on specimens must be marked "Isolation."

If it becomes necessary for laboratory personnel to enter an isolation room, standard isolation procedures must be followed by the technician in regard to himself and his equipment.

If laboratory assistants collect blood, they must follow the precedure for collection of specimens in isolation.

Proper precautions must be taken by laboratory personnel, especially those working with blood, urine, or cultures taken from patients having a communicable disease or infection.

PROCEDURE

Single urine specimens

1. Place clean bottle, label, and cap on isolation cart outside the room.
2. Wash hands; don gown, and mask if indicated.
3. Bring specimen bottle into the bathroom and place it on a paper towel.
4. Obtain specimen according to routine.
5. Pour urine into graduate pitcher and from the pitcher into the specimen bottle until it is half full. Do not contaminate the outside of the container.
6. Measure remainder of urine if necessary, and discard.
7. Wash hands, remove gown and discard in hamper, and rewash hands.
8. Take specimen out of the room and apply a cap and label. Place specimen container in a paper bag, seal with tape, and place in the proper pickup area.

Twenty-four-hour urine specimen. Units without specimen refrigerators may use a basin or pail of ice in the dirty utility room. Care must be taken that contents of the jug or disposable container are not discarded. The outside wrapper of the jug or disposable container should be covered with a plastic bag, secured by tying top of bag at mouth of jug or disposable container with a rubber band or string. Patient's name, room number, and "24-hour urine—isolation" should be marked on the plastic bag. The jug or disposable container is then placed in a basin of ice each time the patient voids during the 24-hour period.

1. Wash hands.
2. Take jug or disposable container from the refrigerator or ice-filled basin. (Containers removed from the ice should be dried with a paper towel.)
3. Take the container and four clean paper towels to the door of the patient's room.
4. Place towels on the floor to the right of the patient's door. Place the jug or container on towels. Remove caps from jugs or if disposable container is used, open one end.
5. Don gown.
6. Collect urine specimen, following the procedure for collecting a single urine specimen. If intake and output are being observed, record the amounts on the intake and output sheet outside the patient's room.
7. Take the urine specimen in graduate pitcher to the doorway of the room. Pour it carefully into the jug or container. Do not spill.
8. Rinse bedpan or urinal and the graduate pitcher and return them to the proper places.

9. Wash hands; remove gown and discard in patient's hamper.
10. Replace cap on jug. Take jug or disposable container to the proper place.
11. Discard paper towels in the waste container.
12. At the end of the 24-hour period, place jug of urine in a paper bag. Mark bag "Isolation—24-hour urine" and send to laboratory.

Stool

1. Place specimen container, cover, label, and tongue blades on the isolation cart outside the room.
2. Wash hands; don gown, mask, and gloves as indicated.
3. Take specimen container and tongue blades into the bathroom and place on paper towels.
4. Use tongue blades to transfer specimen to container. Do not contaminate specimen.
5. Wrap tongue blades in a paper towel and discard into wastebasket.
6. Clean bedpan and return to proper place.
7. Wash hands, remove gown, and repeat hand washing.
8. Take specimen out of the room. Apply cover and label with identification and the word "Isolation."
9. Place in paper bag marked "Isolation," close the bag, attach requisition form, and send to laboratory.

Blood

1. Check information on instruction card on door.
2. Leave laboratory tray on shelf of isolation cart in the corridor. Place two paper towels on the cart to receive contaminated tube specimens, and small plastic bag for slides.
3. Wash hands.
4. Put on gown before entering room, and gloves and/or mask if indicated.
5. Take only necessary equipment into the room from the tray.
6. Take two paper towels from the isolation cart and place them on the patient's overbed table. Equipment is placed on the paper towels; do not place equipment anywhere else in the room.
7. Draw blood and leave tubes in the room.
8. Wash hands.
9. Remove gown, mask, and gloves. Place gown in hamper, and place mask and gloves in wastebasket.

10. Wrap contaminated tubes and equipment in a paper towel. Leave the tourniquet in the room. Take the paper towels outside the room and put the slides in a small plastic bag.
11. Wash hands. (Do not contaminate clothes.)
12. Spray tubes, equipment, and outside plastic bag with disinfectant until wet. Place tubes and plastic bag with slides in the laboratory basket and allow to dry.

Equipment

POLICY. All equipment, including wheelchairs and stretchers, touched by personnel after touching the patient should be cleaned and sprayed with disinfectant before being used for another patient.

For double bagging of isolation equipment, all soiled equipment that is to be transported by cart to central service must first be double bagged. A list of all equipment that is placed inside the bag is essential to central service personnel, who must identify the articles in order to package them properly for sterilization.

CAUTION: *Paper* bags are used for *steam* sterilization. *Plastic* bags are used for *gas* sterilization.

The *objectives* of proper handling of contaminated equipment are (1) to protect personnel and the environment from cross contamination during the packaging of isolation items as they are prepared for sterilization and until sterilization is completed in central service and (2) to prevent these items from being destroyed by improper sterilization due to inadequate or nonexistent identification on the bags.

PROCEDURE

1. *Before entering the room:* Wash hands and put on gown. Take two paper towels, pen, and paper for listing equipment, and a paper or plastic bag (depending on the type of sterilization), into the room.
2. *Inside the room:* To provide an aseptic area for making the list, place the paper towels on the bedside stand and place the sheet of paper on the paper towels.
3. Make the list while hands are still clean. Include diagnosis and room number.
4. *Before sending the bag to central service:* Drain all solutions and rinse equipment well before bagging, including bottles used in suction apparatus, Aqua-Pak machines, and oxygen bottles.
5. Discard all sponges and trash from trays, and throw all linen into contaminated linen hamper.
6. Discard all rubber tubing and plastic connectors.
7. Be sure items are dry before placing them in the bag.

8. After all items have been bagged, fold the edge of the bag twice.
9. At the doorway, the contaminated bag is placed in a clean bag held by an assistant outside the room.
10. The assistant folds the top of the second bag and seals it with masking tape, and tapes the list to the bag. Do not contaminate the list when removing it from the room.
11. Mark the bag "Isolation" and place the bag in the central service pickup.
12. Anything that cannot be transported by cart must be decontaminated on the unit. In the room wash the equipment with disinfectant soap and rinse thoroughly. Spray cart wheels when removing equipment to central service pickup area. Place the following note on the equipment: "Isolation—decontaminated on unit."

Steam sterilization

POLICY. Items made of glass, metal, or stainless steel, including all blue nonmetal bedside utensils, bedpans, washbasins, and emesis basins, can safely be steam-sterilized.

Use double-bagging procedure, with *paper* bags only. Never use one paper bag and one plastic bag.

Remove caps from all glass bottles to prevent explosion in the autoclave.

PROCEDURE (central service personnel)
1. Take double paper bag marked "Isolation." Check the list on the outside of the bag to make certain that all items can be steam sterilized.
2. Place in the section of central service that is reserved for items to be sterilized.
3. Remove from plastic bag and process according to the procedure of each article.

Gas sterilization

POLICY. Gas sterilization is used for delicate instruments, oxygen or suction gauges, blood pressure apparatus, stethoscopes, plastic that would melt or be destroyed such as Aqua-Paks, any motors, and sheepskins.

Use double-bagging procedure, with *plastic* bags only.

Remove caps from all glass bottles.

PROCEDURE (central service personnel)
1. All double plastic bags marked "Isolation" will be gas sterilized.
2. Aerate articles as prescribed for the type of article.

3. Remove from plastic bag and process according to the procedure established for each article.

Thermometers

PROCEDURE (central service personnel)

1. Place bags marked "Isolation thermometers" in assigned area.
2. Place a clean towel on the table to protect the table from accidental contamination by a thermometer or packet.
3. Remove lid from pan containing germicidal solution.
4. Don gloves.
5. Open bag and remove thermometer packets one at a time.
6. Put thermometer in germicidal solution and drop empty packet in step-on can.
7. When all thermometers are in germicidal solution, discard gloves in step-on can.
8. Double-bag contents of step-on container. Sterilize and discard in regular trash container. Step-on cans are also sterilized each day.
9. Leave thermometers in germicidal solution for one hour, and then process as for regular thermometers.

Respiratory therapy equipment

PROCEDURE

Nonpiped-in oxygen

1. To introduce oxygen equipment to an isolation room:
   a. Bring an oxygen tank, equipped with oxygen head and/or respiratory equipment, on a carrier to the patient's room, and leave it outside the door.
   b. Wash hands; don gown, and mask if indicated.
   c. Remove tank from carrier and roll it into the room. The carrier remains outside the oxygen setup.
   d. Follow regular procedure for oxygen setup or for giving a respiratory treatment. If it is necessary to leave two or more tanks in the room, the carrier may be included. Equipment remains in the room.
   e. Wash hands; remove gown and discard into hamper.
   f. Rewash hands.
2. For daily care of respiratory therapy equipment:
   a. Spray tank with disinfectant and change equipment daily.
   b. Double-bag in plastic to send to central service for sterilization. Mark "Isolation—return to respiratory therapy."
   c. Replace supplies.

    d. Before removing the empty tank from the room, spray it with disinfectant. If the patient cannot tolerate the spray, wash the tank with disinfectant solution.

3. For terminal cleaning of respiratory therapy equipment:
    a. Don gown.
    b. Wash all large equipment with disinfectant solution, or spray with disinfectant.
    c. Double-bag in plastic bags all equipment to be sterilized (oxygen head, etc.).
    d. Double-bag in *paper* bags all equipment to be steam sterilized.
    e. Wash hands.
    f. Remove gown, wash hands, and send equipment to central service.
    g. After the oxygen tanks (minus gauges) have been terminally cleaned, they are returned to the respiratory therapy storage area. The gauges are double-bagged in plastic bags, marked "Isolation—return to respiratory therapy," and sent to central service.

4. If respiratory therapy equipment cannot be completely decontaminated on the unit, cover with a plastic bag or pillowcase while transferring it to the respiratory therapy storage area.

Piped-in oxygen

1. Bring equipment to the door of the patient's room and wash hands. Don gown and mask if indicated.
2. Follow regular procedure for setting up oxygen or giving respiratory treatment. The equipment is to be left in the room.
3. Wash hands, remove gown, discard gown in hamper, and rewash hands.
4. Daily and terminal cleaning is the same as for nonpiped-in oxygen.

Electrocardiogram equipment
PROCEDURE

1. *Before entering the room:* Wash hands and don gown and mask if indicated. Cover dials of the equipment with a plastic liner and place all necessary supplies on top of the plastic liner. Attach plastic bag on hanger and hang it on the side of the ECG cart where the tracing will fall.
2. *Inside the room:* follow the usual ECG procedure.
3. Wash electrodes. Spray cable and leads with disinfectant and return them to the drawer.
4. Wash hands; then remove tracings from the bag and roll them.

Place them on top of the machine. Discard plastic bag in waste-basket and replace hanger on side of cart.

5. Wash hands. Remove gown and discard in the room hamper.
6. Wash hands and leave the room.
7. Spray sides of cart, hanger, and wheels with disinfectant.

Traction equipment

POLICY. All traction equipment should be cleaned on the unit by unit personnel.

Only clean equipment should be returned to the traction room. Stored equipment should be checked frequently for cleanliness, and cultures should be taken at random once monthly.

All splints should be repadded after each patient's use. Grossly soiled pads that cannot be washed will be discarded. All disposables will be discarded after patient use.

PROCEDURE

Setting up traction

1. Bring equipment to isolation unit.
2. Wash hands; don gown, mask, and gloves if indicated.
3. Take equipment into the room. Set up as specified by the patient's physician.
4. Check patient for pressure areas and general comfort after applying traction.
5. Wash hands. Discard mask and gloves in the wastebasket, and the gown in the linen hamper.
6. Leave room and notify nurse that traction has been set up or applied.

Removing traction

1. Wash hands, don gloves, gown, and mask if indicated.
2. Take all necessary cleaning supplies into the room.
3. Provide a clean area in the room with newspaper.
4. Wash all traction well. Spray with disinfectant and allow to dry for 2 or 3 minutes.
5. Disassemble equipment. Wash any areas not reached with the disinfectant spray.
6. Remove gloves and mask, and discard in wastebasket; discard gown in linen hamper.
7. Wash hands. Remove traction piece by piece to the outside of the room. Do not contaminate.
8. When all traction equipment is removed, discard the newspaper into the wastebasket.
9. Wash hands and take traction to the traction room.

X-ray department: care of patient and equipment

POLICY. All equipment or supplies used by the isolation patient must be kept from contact with others, and when an isolation patient is brought to the x-ray department, protection of other patients and of x-ray person-nel must be considered. However, the technician should not be reluctant in handling the patient, for hands can always be washed after contact with the patient. Technique and medical asepsis should not be so over-emphasized that the technician will forget the patient.

The patient should never be sent to the x-ray department until the technician is ready. When the patient arrives, his x-ray examination should proceed immediately. If he must wait a few minutes, he should wait in an area away from the other patients.

If the disease is airborne spread, it is preferable that the patient be masked to reduce the spread of disease. If the patient is not masked, then masks must be worn by the transporting attendant and all other persons in the department who are in contact with the patient.

PROCEDURE

X-ray room

1. The technician must wear a gown or mask as indicated by category of isolation.
2. The table must be protected by a clean sheet.
3. If the technician has been contaminated in any way, he must not touch the x-ray machine until his hands have been washed. It is wise to have two technicians available so that one of them can stay "clean."
4. The chair or stretcher in which the patient is brought to the x-ray room must be covered with a clean sheet. The patient side of the sheet is considered contaminated; the underside, which touches the chair or stretcher, is not considered contaminated. Do not let the contaminated side touch the x-ray table. If the sheet becomes wet, it is entirely contaminated.
5. The transportation attendant must wear a gown if he is in direct contact with the patient, such as assisting the patient to the x-ray table. After contact the attendant must change gowns and wash hands before leaving the area.

Nonportable equipment

1. Wash hands and take all unnecessary supplies out of the room.
2. Drape the x-ray table and place a pillow under the drape.
3. Don gown, and mask if indicated, and follow regular x-ray proce-dure.
4. Wash hands and discard gown in the isolation bag.

5. Discard all linen from the table into the red isolation bag. Do not contaminate the outside of the bag.
6. Double-bag disposable supplies, mark "Isolation," and discard in the trash container.
7. Clean nondisposable equipment and supplies and double-bag them to be sent to central service for sterilization. Rinse barium enema equipment with water before bagging.
8. If the x-ray table, stool, and equipment becomes contaminated during the filming, they must be thoroughly scrubbed with a disinfectant or with soap and water.
9. The contaminated technician or others who were in contact with the patient must wash hands and arms thoroughly under running water.
10. Notify the housekeeping service to clean the x-ray room.

Portable x-ray unit

1. Wash hands; don gown, and mask if indicated.
2. Take only the necessary equipment into the room. Place cassettes in individual pillowcases before entering the room.
3. Use regular x-ray procedure established for portable x-ray unit, with the exception that the cassettes are covered.
4. Wash hands. An assistant outside the room may take the cassette after it is removed from the pillow case.
5. Remove gown and discard pillowcases and gowns in the patient's hamper.
6. Push equipment into the corridor and wash hands.
7. Wipe the equipment, including the electrical cord, with alcohol.

Portable x-ray unit in surgery

1. Bring clean portable x-ray unit to surgery.
2. Wash hands. Don mask, gown, and disposable boots before entering the surgical area with the machine.
3. Terminal cleaning of portable equipment must be done before leaving the area.
4. Remove gown and mask.
5. Wash hands.

Code-arrest cart (cardiac resuscitation)

POLICY. The code-arrest cart must be taken into an isolation room when necessary. After use, the cart must be cleaned thoroughly and restocked with all necessary supplies.

PROCEDURE

1. When code arrest is terminated, the *respiratory therapist* will double-bag, in plastic, all respiratory supplies. Mark outside of bag clearly: "Isolation—return to respiratory therapy"; send bags to central service for gas sterilization.
2. *Nursing service personnel* will observe the following procedure:
   a. Remove all pharmacy and central service supplies from the cart drawers.
   b. Double-bag in *paper* all supplies for *steam* sterilization, and list contents on outside of the bag.
   c. Double-bag in *plastic* all supplies to be *gas* sterilized.
   d. Double-bag in *plastic* all medication and I.V. bottles, mark outside of bags "Isolation," and take the bags to pharmacy (medications are not sent by a messenger).
   e. Discard towels from drawers into isolation hamper.
   f. Completely wash cart, drawers, and equipment that can be washed with disinfectant; spray equipment that cannot be washed, using a disinfectant.
   g. Replace clean towels in all drawers and notify pharmacy and respiratory therapy storage unit that the cart is ready to be restocked.
   h. When the cart has been restocked it is returned to the proper unit.

Transportation of the isolation patient

PROCEDURE

1. Drape a sheet over the stretcher or wheelchair. The entire area that touches the bed or patient should be covered.
2. Don gown, mask, gloves as indicated. For respiratory isolation, mask the patient. If the patient is able to use tissues, instruct him in their proper use and provide both tissues and a disposable bag. No mask need be worn by the patient if he takes these precautions. (Transportation attendants need not wear masks or gowns if patient is masked [respiratory] and no direct handling of patient is necessary.)
3. Put a clean gown on the patient and assist him to the stretcher or wheelchair. Avoid touching uncovered portion of the vehicle. Patient's hands should be kept under the sheet at all times. Fasten stretcher or wheelchair straps over the clean sheet.
4. Check the chart cover for isolation label.
5. Report to the department or unit receiving the patient that the patient is from isolation. State the category of isolation and the room number.

6. When transportation of patient is completed, place linen in the patient's isolation linen hamper and spray vehicle with disinfectant.

Terminal cleaning of the isolation room

POLICY. Each isolation room must have its own cleaning equipment. If the patient is found to be free of infection and is removed from isolation (alert category), terminal cleaning is not necessary.

To protect the health of the men who clean the air-conditioning units, they must wear masks and gowns. Masks should be changed as often as necessary during this procedure.

Depending on the individual hospital's procedures, nursing personnel may assist in terminal cleaning of an isolation room. Nursing procedures usually include stripping the bed, double-bagging linen, washing and rinsing bedside utensils, and preparing equipment for sterilization.

Equipment for cleaning the room is on a special isolation cleaning cart outside the patient's room. The mop handle, mop bucket, and a small plastic bucket that was used while the room was occupied is used for the terminal cleaning. A clean mop is used each time a room is cleaned.

Housekeeping personnel wear a gown, mask, and gloves only as indicated. However, if they feel more comfortable wearing full protective garb, they should be allowed to do so.

PROCEDURE

Initial cleaning by housekeeping personnel

1. Before entering the room observe the following procedure:
    a. Wash hands, wrists, and forearms thoroughly with germicidal soap.
    b. Put on gown, mask, cap, and rubber gloves as indicated.
    c. Germicidal solution (2½ ounces), germicidal detergent (1¾ ounces), and scouring powder are brought into the room in disposable paper cups.
2. In the room observe the following procedure:
    a. Fill the plastic bucket with 1 gallon of water and add the germicidal detergent. Fill the mop bucket with 2 gallons of water and add the germicidal solution.
3. Beds
    a. Strip beds. Do not shake the linen but fold it inward to make a bundle and place it with the other soiled linen in the isolation hamper.
    b. Double-bag separately: all rubber sheets, plastic mattress or pillow covers, and blankets made of acrylic fiber or any ma-

terial that fades. Mark the outside of the bag "Isolation" and attach a list of the contents.

    c. Spray and remove the mattress outside the door. The mattress is taken to the housekeeping department, where it is disinfected, aired, and kept for two weeks before being used by another patient.

    d. Spray and scrub the entire bed. Use a small nylon or wire brush soaked in germicidal solution for the small crevices, springs, narrow holes, corners, casters, braces, etc.

4. Wastebaskets

    a. Empty ashtrays into plastic-lined wastebaskets. Remove plastic liners, close them with a pliable red wire tie, and place them near the door. Leave one bag open to dispose of any waste materials left in the room.

    b. Clean the wastebaskets inside and out with germicidal solution and replace plastic liner.

5. Cleaning equipment

    a. Wash and rinse silverware, bedside utensils, and wash-basins that can be steam sterilized, and place in double paper bags. List contents on the outside of the outer bag.

    b. Wash and rinse Aqua-Paks, motors, Biffy brush container, and anything that must be gas-sterilized; place in double plastic bags (this is usually the responsibility of the nurse's aides).

    c. Large equipment must be decontaminated on the unit and marked as such.

6. Telephone

    a. Thoroughly clean crevices, dial, earpiece, and mouthpiece.

    b. Wipe dry and spray with disinfectant spray.

7. Furniture

    a. Spray all furniture with germicidal detergent solution.

    b. Clean inside of drawers and legs, as well as outside area. Be sure all corners and crevices are cleaned.

    c. Clean underside of the furniture, cleaning excessively soiled areas with a brush. Pay special attention to knobs of television set.

8. Windows

    a. Clean inside of all windows.

    b. Remove cubicle curtains and place them in the isolation laundry hamper if they are not disposable. Wash all rods.

    c. Use a stiff brush soaked in germicidal solution to clean crevices.

d. Clean the window curtains by washing both sides with germicidal solution.

9. Floor lamps and wall lamps
   a. Scrub all lamps and wipe clean.
   b. Scrub base of lamp with nylon brush soaked in germicidal solution.
10. Ceiling and walls
    a. Wash ceiling and walls, using wall-washing kit with the proper germicidal solution.
    b. Disassemble and clean all vents. Do not allow excess water to run behind tile.
11. Bathroom
    a. Clean walls and ceiling thoroughly, making sure all corners and crevices are cleaned.
    b. Clean door and hinges.
    c. Clean commode. Scrub inside of toilet bowl with bowl cleanser, using swab brush. Allow cleanser to remain in the bowl for 3 or 4 minutes. Clean particularly well under the rim. Flush toilet, using swab brush to thoroughly rinse the bowl.
    d. Thoroughly clean and scour all pipes under the sinks. Clean and shine all faucets.
    e. Clean sinks with germicidal solution and scouring powder. Follow with germicidal rinse.
    f. Scrub bathtub with abrasive powder and rinse thoroughly.
    g. Thoroughly clean the shower room from top to bottom. Scrub the walls with proper germicidal solution.
12. Floor
    a. Clean floor with the proper germicidal solution. Scrub all mop boards.
    b. Use a putty knife and steel wool to clean very soiled surfaces.
    c. Generously spray water on the floor until the floor is well covered; let water stand for 5 minutes. Remove the water with a wet vacuum pickup.
13. After the floor is dry, replace furniture. Spray all furniture with disinfectant spray.
14. Place a clean mattress on the bed and make the bed.
15. Hang clean cubicle curtains.

Final cleaning and inspection

1. Wash all cleaning equipment and plastic containers with germicidal solution.
2. Dispose of germicidal solution in toilet bowl.

3. Remove mop and place it into a plastic bag for removal to the laundry area. Tie it closed with a red tie. Double-bag all trash, disposables, and linen, assisted by a person outside the door.
4. Remove gloves and mask, and deposit them in the final trash bag.
5. Untie gown strings. Deposit gown in the hamper provided.
6. Before leaving, survey the room to be sure that all furniture is in place and all cleaning has been accomplished.
7. Wash hands, wrists, and forearms thoroughly with germicidal solution.
8. Notify the supervisor that the room is ready for culturing.

Cultures

The following are usually the responsibility of trained housekeeping supervisors:

1. Pick up culture plates from the microbiology laboratory.
2. Take cultures before any one enters the newly cleaned room.
3. After cultures have been taken, notify the nursing station that the room is ready for occupancy.

Cleaning of multiple-occupancy units with probable contamination. When a patient is admitted to a multiple-occupancy room and, after admission, it is determined that the patient has a possible communicable disease and is subsequently transferred to the isolation wing, the cleaning procedure will be as follows:

1. Inform cleaning personnel to take isolation cleaning precautions.
2. Seal off contaminated area within the room.
3. Remove bed linen and cubicle curtains, place into isolation bag, and remove to soiled linen area.
4. Wash mattress and remove to housekeeping storage area.
5. Wash walls, bed, furniture, and fixtures with germicidal solution.
6. Place clean mattress on the bed and hang freshly laundered cubicle curtains.
7. Thoroughly mop floor area, following the isolation mopping procedure.
8. While in the patient's room, do not disturb the other patients and do not discuss the isolation procedures within hearing distance of the other patients.
9. Take cultures before room is released for new occupant (culturing is an individual hospital preference).

Care of body after death
PROCEDURE

1. Don gown, mask, and gloves if indicated.
2. Prepare body according to hospital procedure. Confine any drain-

ing area with dressings. Identification tags must be stamped with "Isolation" and the type of isolation category the patient was in.

3. Drape stretcher with a sheet.
4. Place the patient on stretcher and cover with another sheet. Isolation tape should be applied to the shroud. Fasten the stretcher straps over the clean sheet. Avoid touching the clean sheet with the gown.
5. Wash hands; remove gown, mask, and gloves.
6. Wash hands again.
7. Transport patient to the morgue and place the body in the proper compartment.
8. Strip the cart and place the linen in the isolation bag. Wash the stretcher with soap and water and spray with disinfectant.
9. Wash hands.
10. The patient's clothing is given to the family or taken to the proper place, in a bag marked with the patient's name, unit, and "Isolation." Patient's clothing should be listed before bagging, and the list stapled to the outside of the bag.

Discharge of patient from isolation
PROCEDURE
Discharge home

1. Don gown if necessary.
2. Cut off identification band.
3. Instruct patient to bathe, and shampoo hair according to physician's orders.
4. Place a clean sheet over the bed and place the patient's clean clothes on the sheet.
5. Instruct the patient to dress.
6. Wash hands, discard gown, rewash hands.
7. Discharge patient according to hospital procedure.
8. Request terminal cleaning of the room.

Transfer to another room

1. Don gown.
2. Remove soiled top linen from the bed.
3. Place a clean sheet over the bed.
4. Cut off patient's identification band. Instruct patient to take a complete bath or shower, and shampoo hair according to physician's orders.
5. Put a clean gown on the patient and replace the identification band with a new one.
6. Transfer patient to the newly assigned room.

7. All personal items taken by the patient to the new room must be sprayed with disinfectant or washed in disinfectant soap and water.
8. Clothes sent home with relatives are to be cleaned with disinfectant or aired in the sun for 8 hours.
9. Request terminal cleaning of the contaminated room.

Removal from isolation category but remaining in same room

1. Don gown. Remove patient's identification band.
2. Instruct the patient to take a complete bath and shampoo hair according to physician's orders. Provide a clean gown for the patient.
3. If the patient is able to bathe without assistance, strip the bed, wash, and remake the bed with clean linen while the patient is in the bathroom. Do not shake the linen while placing it in the isolation hamper.
4. If a bed bath is necessary, care must be taken to remove linen without contamination and to wash the bed thoroughly.
5. All personal articles are washed or sprayed with disinfectant.
6. Room is cleaned according to terminal procedure.
7. Wash hands.
8. Place a clean identification band on patient's arm.
9. Remove gown and wash hands.

High-risk areas
Intensive Care Unit (ICU)

POLICY. Since ICU is a high-risk area, all ICU patients having communicable diseases or infection must be located in *rooms,* not cubicles.

The *isolation technique* is chosen according to category of the disease and must be followed.

The unit must be terminally *cleaned* after patient's discharge if the disease or infection was communicable.

Handwashing before and after patient care or handling of contaminated equipment is mandatory.

All *personnel* working in the area must be free from communicable respiratory disease or any overt wound infection.

Strict asepsis is mandatory for *tracheostomy care,* and for *urinary care* and irrigations.

All dressings must be double bagged in plastic and discarded in the dressing container.

Emergency room

POLICY. A special room away from the emergency room proper should be used in the case of infected wounds (incision and drainage).

Instruments must be rinsed with running water, autoclaved for 7 minutes, and then cleaned in the regular manner.

Linen must be placed in a red bag; disposable supplies must be bagged and discarded properly.

Tables are wiped with alcohol or sprayed with disinfectant.

PROCEDURE

Care of patient with communicable disease

1. If the presence of disease (for example, meningitis) is known in advance, remove all unnecessary furniture and supplies from the emergency room to be used by this patient.
2. When the disease is known or suspected, personnel must wear a gown and mask while treating the patient.
3. *If the patient is admitted to the hospital,* all precautions must be taken to prevent the spread of infection or disease before the patient is transported to the assigned area. Mask or gown the patient as indicated. To alert the unit, attach an isolation sticker to the front of the envelope containing emergency room reports and physician's orders.
4. Place clothing in a plastic bag and send it home with the family or to the patient's room.

Cleaning the emergency room

1. Call cleaning service to terminally clean the room.
2. Place all linen in a red bag.
3. Hang clean curtains.
4. Clean stretcher and pillow with alcohol and spray with disinfectant. Clean and spray all nondisposable equipment that cannot be autoclaved.

Recovery room

POLICY. Patients from respiratory isolation are not admitted to the recovery room but are returned to their room immediately after surgery unless this is contraindicated because of the patient's critical condition. Then precautions must be set up in the recovery area. A recovery room nurse should accompany the patient to his room and remain with him until he reacts and his vital signs are stable.

Patients who have undergone such procedures as an incision and drainage of a rectal abscess or a Bartholin's gland cyst are admitted to the recovery room but require special handling. The patient is placed in an area away from other patients, and one nurse is responsible for his care while he remains.

Special precautions are taken in handling soiled linen and dressings.

Careful handwashing by the attending nurse is carried out to prevent cross contamination.

Surgery (septic cases)

POLICY. A safe environment must be maintained to prevent cross contamination from septic to clean cases. The newest trend is to treat every patient as a possible dirty or septic case and act accordingly.

Types of septic cases include local abscesses, wounds with frank pus, tuberculosis and other active infectious diseases, draining infected wounds, gas gangrene, and tetanus.

Areas and equipment considered contaminated include the perimeter of the operating room table, other parts of room where there may be spillage of contaminated material; members of the sterile team until they have discarded gowns, gloves, caps, masks, and shoe covers; anesthesia equipment and personnel; and the stretcher used to transport the patient.

PROCEDURE

Prior to surgery (circulator with no gown or gloves)

1. Assemble all supplies and equipment.
2. Move unnecessary furniture and equipment into corridor.
3. Bring into the room only necessary supplies.
4. For known septic cases, place floor mat saturated with disinfectant outside operating room door and remove after case cleanup.

During surgery (circulator)

1. Admit only necessary personnel. Control traffic in and out of room.
2. Strict adherence to good aseptic principles must be followed when using room supplies. It is preferable for someone outside the room to obtain supplies that are not located in the room.
3. Pick up contaminated sponges with ring forceps.
4. Watch closely for any lapses in sterile technique by physicians or nurses.

After surgery (circulator or scrub nurse)

1. Wearing mask, gloves, and shoe covers, discard disposable materials into plastic bags. (All surgical personnel and physicians must remove masks, gowns, gloves, and shoe covers before leaving the surgery room.)
2. Wash all instruments and autoclave them.
3. Scrub all articles intolerant of heat and soak in disinfectant. The basin must be covered during the soaking.
4. Empty solution into utility hopper and flush. Follow this with disinfectant.

5. Discard all linen into contaminated linen hamper.
6. Wash all furniture well with disinfectant.
7. Discard gloves, mask, and shoe covers after the room is completely clean. Wash hands and change into clean scrub gown. Rewash hands.

Isolation nursery

POLICY. The purpose of a special routine is to prevent cross contamination of babies or of their immediate crib environment.

Flashlight, otoscope, and stethoscope remain in the isolation nursery.

Each baby must be in a separate nursery unless other babies have the same type of infection or disease. An Isolette may act as an isolation unit provided that only the armholes are used.

Babies in the isolation nursery should not go out to their mothers.

PROCEDURE

1. Scrub hands; don gown and mask if indicated. Use gown only once.
2. Care for baby and then scrub hands.
3. Discard gown into hamper in isolation nursery and mask into wastebasket; scrub hands again.
4. Linen must be double bagged. Blankets, shirts, sheets, and gowns do not have to be separated. Disposable diapers should be used.
5. Nursery is terminally cleaned after all babies are discharged. The incubator or Isolette is cleaned by nursery personnel and then gas sterilized.
6. At the discretion of the physician, babies in isolation nursery will be moved to full-term nursery if culture and/or gastric contents fail to demonstrate infection.

CATEGORIES OF ISOLATION

The practice of isolation is complicated, time-consuming, costly, and inconvenient. It is a continuous process of modification, since the length of the patient's stay in isolation is governed by mode of transmission, virulence of the disease, and the incubation period. Research is constantly discovering new facts on communicable diseases that tend to shorten the known period of communicability, thereby decreasing the period of isolation.

The basic purpose of isolation is to confine the infectious agent to a restricted area until its danger of spread has been controlled.

In order to initiate proper isolation precautions for a particular type of infection or disease, categories of isolation should be established. Since variations in isolation methods are expected among hospitals, the isolation system detailed here is intended as a guide only.

To accommodate the differences in the epidemiology of infectious diseases, classification has been limited to six categories: alert, enteric, respiratory, strict, wound and skin, and reverse. Each category is identified with a color code, which is employed each time that particular category of isolation is utilized in any area of the hospital.

LIST OF GENERAL DISEASES—CATEGORY AND DURATION

	Key	Color
A	Alert	White
E	Enteric	Green
N	None required	None
RV	Reverse	Blue
S	Strict	Yellow
WS	Wound and skin	Pink
R	Respiratory	Red
BP	Blood precautions	None
SE	Secretion precautions	None
EX	Excretion precautions	None

DURATION OF ISOLATION OR PRECAUTION

CN	Until off antibiotics and until culture is negative
DH	Duration of hospitalization
DI	Duration of illness (with wounds or lesions, DI means until they stop draining)
U	Until 24 hours after initiation of effective therapy
*	Specific precautions listed for disease

	CATEGORY OF ISOLATION		
DISEASE	**Adults**	**Children**	**Duration**
Abscess or boil	WS	WS	DI
Actinomycosis (draining lesions)	SE	SE	DI
Agranulocytosis	RV	RV	DI
Anthrax (cutaneous)	SE	SE	CN
Anthrax (inhalation)	S	S	DI
Anticancer therapy (immunosuppressive therapy)	RV	RV	DH
Arthropod-borne viral encephalitides			
Eastern equine encephalitis			
Western equine encephalitis			
St. Louis encephalitis	N	N	
Arthropoid-borne viral fevers			
Yellow fever			
Hemolytic-uremic syndrome	BP	BP	DI
Ascariasis	N	N	DI
Aspergillosis	N	N	
Blastomycosis—North American	N	N	
Brucellosis (undulant fever, Malta fever)			
Draining lesions	SE	SE	DI

Continued.

DISEASE	CATEGORY OF ISOLATION		
	Adults	Children	Duration
Burns, infected (staphylococci or streptococci)	WS	WS	DI
Burns, uninfected	RV	RV	
Candidiasis (moniliasis, thrush)	N	A	DI
*In pediatrics, special nipple and bottle precautions			
Cat-scratch fever (benign inoculation)	N	N	
Chancroid (ulcus molle, soft chancre)	N	N	
Chickenpox (varicella)	R	R	*
*For 7 days after eruption appears			
Cholera	E	E	DI
Coccidioidomycosis (valley fever)			
Pneumonia	N	N	
Draining wound	WS	WS	DI
Conjunctivitis, acute bacterial (sore eyes, pinkeye)	WS & SE	WS & SE	U
Conjunctivitis, gonorrheal (ophthalmia neonatorum)	WS	WS	U
Conjunctivitis, inclusion			
Neonatal inclusion blennorrhea			
Paratrachoma			
Swimming pool conjunctivitis	N	N	DI
Cryptococcosis (torulosis, European blastomycosis)	WS	WS	DI
Dermatitis (uninfected)	RV	RV	DI
Diarrheas (possibly infectious)	E	E	
Diphtheria	S	S	*
*Until two cultures taken at least 24 hours apart after cessation of antibiotic therapy for the nose and throat are negative for *Corynebacterium diphtheriae*			
Echinococcosis (hydatidosis)	N	N	
Encephalitis, arthropod-borne	N	N	
Encephalomyelitis			
Venezuelan equine encephalomyelitis	N	N	
Enterobiasis (pinworm disease, oxyuriasis)	N	N	
*Linen precautions			
Enteroviral infections (viral diarrhea)	E	E	DI
Escherichia coli enteropathogenic gastroenteritis	E	E	DI
Fevers of undetermined origin	A	A	
Furunculosis	WS	WS	DI
Gas gangrene	WS	WS	
Surgical area	S	S	
Gonorrhea	WS	WS	U
Gonorrheal ophthalmia neonatorum (acute conjunctivitis of the newborn)	WS & SE	WS & SE	U
Granuloma inguinale (donovanosis, granuloma venereum)	WS & SE	WS & SE	DI

DISEASE	CATEGORY OF ISOLATION		
	Adults	**Children**	**Duration**
Hepatitis, infectious			
Epidemic hepatitis (epidemic jaundice)			
Catarrhal jaundice	E	E	DH
Possible hepatitis	E	E	
Hepatitis, serum (homologous serum jaundice)	E	E	DH
Herpangina	E	E	DH
Herpes simplex (neonatal)	S	S	DI
Herpes zoster, eruptive	WS & R	WS & R	DI
Histoplasmosis	N	N	
Hookworm disease (ancylostomiasis, uncinariasis)	N	N	
Immunosuppressive therapy (at physician's request)	R	R	DI
Influenza	A & SE	A & SE	DI
Keratoconjunctivitis, infectious			
Epidemic keratoconjunctivitis			
Infectious punctate keratitis	WS & SE	WS & SE	DI
Leprosy	N	N	
Leptospirosis (Weil's disease, canicola fever, hemorrhagic jaundice, Fort Bragg fever)	E	E	DH
Leukemias and leukopenia	R	R	DI
Listeriosis (meningitis)	N	N	
Other	SE	SE	DI
Lymphocytic choriomeningitis	N	N	
Lymphogranuloma venereum (lymphogranuloma inguinale, climatic Bubo)	SE	SE	DI
Malaria	BP	BP	DH
Measles (morbilli, rubeola)			
Encephalitis	N	N	
Exanthem subitum (roseola infantum)	N	N	*
*For 7 days after rash appears			
Rubella (congenital syndrome in newborn to 1 year of age)	S	S	DI
Rubella	R	R	*
*For 5 days after rash appears			
Melioidosis	S	S	DI
Meningitis (nonbacterial and bacterial)			
Meningococcic meningitis (viral meningitis)	R	R	U
Serous meningitis	R&E SE	R&E SE	DH
Undiagnosed meningitis (until diagnosis is proved)	R	R	
Mononucleosis, infectious (glandular fever, monocytic angina)	N	N	
Mumps (infectious parotitis)	R	R	*
*For 9 days after onset of swelling			
Nocardiosis, with draining lesions	WS & SE	WS & SE	DI

Continued.

DISEASE	CATEGORY OF ISOLATION		
	Adults	Children	Duration
Plague			
Pneumonic	S	S	CN
Bubonic	S	S	CN
Pleurodynia (Bornholm disease, epidemic myalgia)	E	E	DH
*Nose and throat discharge precautions also necessary; causative agent, Coxsackie virus, group B)			
Pneumonias			
Beta hemolytic streptococcus, group A	S	S	DI
Mycoplasmal pneumonia (primary atypical pneumonia, Eaton agent pneumonia)	SE	SE	DI
Pneumococcal pneumonia	N	A	DI
Staphylococcus, coagulase-positive form	S	S	DI
Virus pneumonia, except influenza	N	A	DI
Poliomyelitis (infantile paralysis)	E	E	DH
Psittacosis (ornithosis)	SE	SE	DI
Q fever	SE	SE	DI
Rabies (hydrophobia)	S	S	DI
Rashes (suspicious)	A	A	
Rat-bite fever			
Spirillum minus disease (sodoku)	N	N	
Streptobacillus moniliformis disease (Haverhill fever)	N	N	
Relapsing fever	N	N	
Renal failure (acute)	RV	RV	DI
Respiratory disease, acute viral			
Acute febrile respiratory disease	SE	SE & A	DI
Common cold	SE	SE	DI
Rheumatic fever	N	N	
Rickettsialpox (vesicular rickettsiosis)	N	N	
Ringworm (dermatophytosis, dermatomycosis, tinea)			
Ringworm of body	N	N	
Ringworm of foot	N	N	
Ringworm of nails	N	N	
Ringworm of scalp	N	WS	DI
*Use linen precautions on all types			
Roseola infantum	N	N	
Rubella (congenital syndrome, newborn to 1 year of age)	S	S	DH
Rubella (German measles)	R	R	*
*For 5 days after rash appears			
Rubeola (measles)	R	R	*
*For 7 days after eruption appears			
Salmonella gastroenteritis	E	E	DI
Scabies	N	N	
*Linen precaution			

	CATEGORY OF ISOLATION		
DISEASE	**Adults**	**Children**	**Duration**
Scarlet fever (scarlatina)	R	R	
Schistosomiasis (bilharziosis)	N	N	
Shigellosis (bacillary dysentery)	E	E	DI
Smallpox (variola)	S	S	*
*Until all crusts are shed			
Staphylococcal coagulase-positive disease			
Burns	WS	WS	DI
Dermatitis	WS & R	WS & R	DI
Enteritis	E	E	DI
Pemphigus (especially in nursery)	WS & R	WS & R	DI
Pneumonia	R	R	DI
Wounds (move patient from surgical service if possible)	WS & R	WS & R	DI
Streptococcal disease (beta hemolytic streptococcus, group A)			
Abscess	WS & R	WS & R	DI
Burns	WS & R	WS & R	DI
Erysipelas	WS & R	WS & R	
Impetigo	WS & R	WS & R	DI
Pharyngitis	R	R	U
Pneumonia	R	R	DI
Syphilis (primary, secondary)	WS	WS	U
Teniasis and cysticercosis (beef or pork tapeworm disease)	E	E	DI
Tetanus	N	N	
Toxoplasmosis	N	N	
Trachoma	SE	SE	DI
Trichinosis (trichinellosis, trichiniasis)	N	N	
Trichomoniasis	N	N	
Trichuriasis (trichocephaliasis, whipworm disease)	N	N	
Tuberculosis			
Meningitis	N	N	
Meningitis with pulmonary lesion	R	R	*
Pulmonary	R	R	*
*Until effective therapy begins and there is clinical improvement			
Renal (possibly pulmonary)	A	A	
Tularemia	WS	WS	DI
Typhoid fever (enteric fever, typhus abdominalis)	E	E	*
*Until there are three consecutive negative cultures of feces taken 24 hours apart			
Typhus fever, endemic flea-borne (murine typhus)	N	N	
Typhus fever, endemic louse-borne (typhus exanthematicus, classic typhus fever)	N	N	
Vaccinia, generalized and progressive	WS & S	WS & S	DI
Venereal diseases	WS	WS	U

Continued.

DISEASE	CATEGORY OF ISOLATION		
	Adults	Children	Duration
Viral diseases	R	R	DH
Whooping cough (pertussis)	R	R	DH
Wounds			
Possibly staphylococcus-positive wounds or infection caused by beta hemolytic streptococcus, group A, of any wound postoperatively	WS & R	WS & R	DI
Wounds proved to have organisms (other) with much drainage, such as pathogenic *Pseudomonas*	WS & SE	WS & SE	DI

There are two procedures that apply to all categories: handwashing and explaining the meaning of isolation to each patient admitted for any infection or communicable disease. Handwashing is mandatory for all procedures in all categories.

Alert category

The purpose of the alert category of isolation is to provide special precautions to be used when a physician (or nurse with physician's permission) suspects a disease or infection and awaits proof through laboratory test or x-ray examination. This category is an interim one and should be used only for short durations.

COLOR CODE: WHITE
SAMPLE OF ALERT CATEGORY DOOR CARD

VISITORS INQUIRE AT NURSES STATION BEFORE ENTERING ROOM

Gowns, masks, gloves: Worn only when required to protect yourself or others.
Hands: *Everyone* must wash hands *well* with soap and water before entering or leaving room.
Articles: Special precautions for contaminated linen, dressings, feces and urine (for diarrheal problems), and tissue (for respiratory problems).

Note: _____

_____

Diseases that signify use of alert category

1. Diarrheas (nondiagnosed)
2. Fevers of undetermined origin
3. Draining wounds that appear infected.
4. Jaundice (suspicion of hepatitis)

5. Possible tuberculosis (nondiagnosed)
6. Possible meningitis (any communicable disease nondiagnosed)
7. Suspicious rashes of undetermined origin
8. All respiratory diseases not demanding respiratory technique

General comments

1. Initiate precautions according to the route of transmission for the suspected disease. For example, enteric precautions should be used for nondiagnosed diarrheas or possible infectious hepatitis; wound and skin precautions should be initiated for suspicious draining wounds.

2. When tests indicate that the patient has a communicable disease or infection, the physician is notified, the patient is transferred to the indicated category of isolation, and the door card is changed. Terminal disinfection is used after the patient's transfer or discharge.

3. When tests indicate that the patient is not infectious, alert precautions are discontinued and the patient is placed on routine care. General cleaning is done after patient's transfer or discharge.

Major precautions

Room. Private room is desirable if possible. A semiprivate room may be used if necessary; however, exceptional precautions should be taken in a semiprivate room.

Gown, gloves, and mask. Use will depend on the type of illness involved and the cooperativeness of the patient.

Linen. All linen should be double bagged, with a red outer bag. Avoid airborne spread of bacteria by careful handling of linen. Hamper may be left in room if the room is private.

Needles and syringes. In cases of possible hepatitis patients, use needle and syringe precautions listed under the enteric category.

Specimens. No special precautions except for diarrhea or possible hepatitis. Hepatitis patients use technique listed under the enteric category.

Thermometer. Use thermometer precautions listed under the strict category.

Dishes and food. Disposable dishes should be used, and then discarded in a double plastic bag that has been sealed and marked "Isolation" and discarded in the proper container. Utensils are washed after each use, wrapped in a paper towel, and left in the patient's room. Terminal sterilization is done after discharge.

Dressings and tissues. Must be placed in double plastic bag and discarded into the proper container—not in the patient's wastebasket.

Excreta. Special precautions for diarrhea and possible hepatitis problems. Bedpans and urinals must be rinsed well after each use and returned to the patient's bedside. The patient is to have his own toilet or commode.

Transportation. Supply tissues and bag when there is a possibility of tuberculosis or communicable disease. Mask patient if indicated. Inform the department that the patient is in the alert category.

Terminal disinfection. Necessary only if patient's disease or infection proves to be communicable.

Visitors. Limited to two at one time. Gowns are necessary if they are having direct contact with the patient.

Enteric category

The purpose of the enteric category of isolation is to prevent disease that can be transmitted through direct or indirect contact with infected feces, in some instances throat secretions, urine, or heavily contaminated articles. Transmission depends on oral ingestion of the pathogen.

COLOR CODE: GREEN
SAMPLE OF ENTERIC CATEGORY DOOR CARD

VISITORS INQUIRE AT NURSES STATION BEFORE ENTERING ROOM

Gown and gloves: To be worn by all persons handling soiled linen or having direct contact with urine, feces, or articles contaminated with above.

Masks: Not necessary.

Hands: *Everyone* must wash hands *well* with soap and water before leaving unit.

Articles: Special precautions for articles contaminated by feces, urine, or vomitus. Articles are double bagged for terminal sterilization.

Note: _____

_____

Diseases that signify use of enteric category

1. Diarrheas (infectious)
   a. Amebiasis (dysentery)
   b. Bacillary dysentery *(Shigella)*
   c. Enteropathogens *(Escherichia coli)*
   d. Salmonellosis
   e. Staphylococcal enteritis (*Staphylococcus aureus*–positive)
   f. Viral diarrheas (enteroviruses)
2. Diseases with enteric problems
   a. Hepatitis (infectious or serum)
   b. Typhoid fever

General comments

1. Gamma globulin is advised for the following hospital contacts who did not take proper precautions: pregnant nurses or aides, and staff members who received accidental needle punctures in caring for the patient.

2. Handwashing and gown-and-glove technique for excreta are sufficient to control cross contamination. Avoid needle pricks.

Major precautions

Room. Semiprivate room may be used (children must be in a private room). Infected patient must use a commode, which is cleaned well after use and decontaminated before being returned to central service.

Gown, gloves, and mask. Gown and gloves are used for handling all feces, urine, or soiled linen. A mask is not necessary.

Linen. Hamper should be kept in the patient's room. Double-bag technique is used (red bag on outside). Hot-water–soluble bags are preferred, since they may be placed unopened in hospital washing machines. Plastics and blankets are separated from the linen. They should be placed in a double plastic bag and marked "Isolation."

Needles and syringes. Special precautions are taken in cases of hepatitis. Only disposables should be used. They should be carried in a paper towel from the room to the isolation needle-and-syringe box at the nurses station. (Needles should never be left in the patient's room.)

Specimens. Should be placed in sterile, labeled containers and tightly closed. They are then marked "Isolation" and sent to the laboratory.

Sphygmomanometer and stethoscope. No special precautions unless contaminated by excreta.

Thermometer. Electronic or disposable thermometers are preferred. Glass thermometers should be placed soiled end down into their packet and then into a paper bag marked "Isolation." The bag should be sealed and returned to central service on each shift.

Special instruments and trays. Should be rinsed and double bagged. Outer bag is marked "Isolation" and return to central service for sterilization.

Dishes and food. Disposable dishes are preferred. Nothing should be sent to the kitchen until it has been terminally sterilized by central service (for example, nondisposable silverware).

Dressings and tissues. Place in a plastic bag and seal with tape. Discard in dressing container in utility room.

Excreta. Should be flushed down the toilet. Clean the utensils and replace them at bedside. Double-bag for sterilization on patient's discharge and label "Isolation" before sending to central service.

Transportation. No precautions except for incontinent patients. These patients should have a clean sheet and pajamas before transportation. If the patient is incontinent at the time of transportation, the wheelchair or stretcher should be washed and sprayed with a disinfectant after the patient is returned to the unit.

Terminal disinfection. Special care is taken of bathroom and utensils used in elimination. Double-bagging procedure is used for sterilization by central service.

Visitors. Limited to two visitors. They are gowned and must use handwashing procedure.

Respiratory category

The purpose of the respiratory category is to prevent transmission of airborne organisms by means of droplets and droplet nuclei that are coughed, sneezed, or breathed into the environment, or by means of freshly contaminated articles.

COLOR CODE: RED
SAMPLE OF RESPIRATORY CATEGORY DOOR CARD

VISITORS INQUIRE AT NURSES STATION BEFORE ENTERING ROOM

Room:	*Keep door closed* except for entrances and exits of personnel.
Gowns:	Not necessary except when holding infants.
Masks:	Must be worn by all persons entering the room who are susceptible to the disease.
Hands:	Must be washed on entering and leaving room.
Gloves:	Not necessary.
Articles:	Those contaminated with secretion must be disinfected.
Note:	_____
	_____

Diseases that require use of respiratory category

1. Herpes zoster
2. Measles
   a. Rubella
   b. Rubeola
3. Meningococcic meningitis
4. Meningococcemia
5. Chickenpox
6. Mumps
7. Pertussis
8. Tuberculosis

  a. Pulmonary
  b. Sputum positive (or suspect)
9. Venezuelan equine encephalomyelitis

General comments

1. Use of private room, proper handwashing, secretion precautions, and masks is sufficient to prevent transmission of these diseases.

2. Patients with the same disease may stay in the same room if permission is obtained from each patient's physician.

3. In adult areas, a mask is sufficient protection. It must be worn either by the patient or by the person visiting or giving treatment—but preferably by the patient who is spreading the organism. The newest trend in prevention of respiratory disease transmission is toward eliminating the mask by teaching proper tissue technique to patients and personnel. For the care of small children, personnel must wear both mask and gown because of the possibility of drooling by the infant, which soils the uniform of the personnel.

4. The following diseases provide immunity:
    a. Measles (rubeola or rubella). After having disease, the patient acquires permanent immunity. Vaccination provides a two-year immunity.
    b. Mumps. Involvement of both sides confers lifelong immunity. If only one side is involved, it may occur again on one side or both.
    c. Poliomyelitis. Permanent immunity ensues after recovery for the type acquired. Sabin (sugar cube) vaccine confers debatable immunity.
    d. Chickenpox. One attack confers permanent immunity.
    e. Whooping cough (pertussis). Prolonged immunity is acquired after first attack, but diseases may recur in adult.

5. For a patient with herpes zoster it is especially important to isolate him from highly susceptible patients (on steroids, immunosuppressive therapy, etc.).

Major precautions

Room. Private room necessary unless other patient in the same room has the same disease and permission for sharing the room has been obtained from both physicians.

Gown. Need not be worn except when caring for infants-in-arms.

Mask. Must be worn by either patient or personnel. It is preferred that the patient wear the mask. All personnel or visitors must wear a mask if they are susceptible to the disease.

Linen. No special precautions.

Specimens. Must be double bagged and clearly marked if tuberculosis is present. Close-fitting lids must be placed on all specimen containers.

Sphygmomanometer and stethoscope. Left in patient's room during time of admission. It is to be double bagged in plastic and returned to central service at the time of patient's discharge.

Thermometer. Electronic or kit thermometer preferred. Glass thermometer is placed soiled end down in its packet and then in a paper bag marked "Isolation" and sent to central service at the end of each shift.

Dishes. Disposable dishes are preferred.

Dressings and tissues. Must be double bagged in plastic and discarded in proper container.

Excreta. No special precautions except for polio patients.

Transportation. Patient must wear a mask when leaving the room. The person transporting the patient need not wear a mask if the patient is masked.

Terminal disinfection. Good general cleaning, with particular attention to vents and filters. The room should be aired, if possible for 1 or 2 hours before cleaning.

Visitors. Immediate family, two at a time, with instructions about masks given by nursing personnel before room is entered.

Strict category

The purpose of the strict category is to establish special precautions for all highly communicable diseases that produce serious diseases in susceptible individuals. It is designed to control both airborne and contact spread of disease.

COLOR CODE: YELLOW
SAMPLE OF STRICT CATEGORY DOOR CARD

VISITORS INQUIRE AT NURSES STATION BEFORE ENTERING ROOM

Room:	Private room *necessary*. Door must be kept closed.
Gown, mask, gloves:	Must be worn by all persons entering room.
Hands:	Must be washed on entering and leaving room.
Articles:	Must be discarded, or wrapped before being sent to central service for disinfection or sterilization.
Note:	_____
	_____

Diseases that signify use of strict category

1. Anthrax
2. Rabies
3. Diphtheria
4. Plague (bubonic or pneumonic)
5. Pneumonia
   a. Staphylococcus, coagulase-positive
   b. Streptococcus, beta hemolytic, group A
6. Smallpox (see special section on smallpox precautions)
7. Rubella syndrome (congenital—newborn to 1 year of age)
8. Vaccinia
   a. Generalized
   b. Progressive

General comments

1. A private room with connecting toilet facilities is a must. Doors *must* be kept *closed* at all times except for necessary entrances or exits because of the airborne problem of these diseases.

2. *Two* employees are necessary to implement a correct, safe, double-bagging procedure. Double paper bags must be used, and a list of all articles contained in the bag must be placed on the outer bag, which is clearly marked "Isolation."

3. Visitors and equipment are kept to a minimum in the isolation room.

4. Some communicable diseases establish immunity: smallpox confers permanent immunity after recovery, whereas vaccination provides a ten-year immunity.

Major precautions

Room. Private, with separate bathroom facilities. Door is kept closed.

Gown, gloves, and mask. Worn by all persons entering the room.

Linen. Double bags, with red outside bag. Water-soluble bags preferred. Blankets and plastics are placed in separate bags marked "Isolation."

Needles and syringes. Disposable preferred. They are marked and placed in the isolation box for needles and syringes in the nurses station. When the box is full, it should be sealed. Do not leave needles or syringes in the patient's room.

Patient's chart. Must be kept outside isolation room.

Specimens. Place in a tightly closed container and then into a single paper bag labeled "Isolation."

Sphygmomanometer and stethoscope. Should be left in the room.

Thermometer. Electronic or disposable thermometers recommended. At the end of each shift, glass thermometers are to be placed soiled end down into packet, placed in a paper bag marked "Isolation," and sent to central service for sterilization. Disposable thermometers are destroyed after discharge.

Special instruments or trays. Follow double-bagging procedure.

Books, magazines, and letters. If visibly soiled with potentially infective excretions or secretions, they should be disinfected or destroyed. There are special precautions for smallpox.

Clothing and personal effects. Should be double bagged and sent home.

Dishes. Should be disposable, and discarded on the unit. They should never be sent to the kitchen, even if they are double bagged. If silverware is not disposable, it should be cleaned after each meal and wrapped in a paper towel for sterilization. When the patient is discharged, silverware should be double bagged, marked "Isolation," and sent to central service to be sterilized before being returned to the kitchen.

Dressings and tissues. Dressings should be handled with surgical instruments. All soiled dressings are sealed in a double plastic bag and discarded in a covered container marked "Dressings" in the soiled utility room.

Concurrent cleaning. Each room has its own cleaning equipment. Regular procedures for cleaning should be followed, except that a gown, mask, and gloves are worn. (Cleaning compound is not left in room.)

Terminal disinfection. Nursing service personnel should notify the environmental service that the room is empty and needs terminal disinfection. Procedure for terminal cleaning is then used.

Visitors. Must follow the procedure explained by nursing personnel. Only two persons at a time may visit, and they must wear a gown, mask, and gloves.

Smallpox precautions

Special precautions for smallpox are necessary because of the virulence of the disease in unvaccinated persons and the stability of the virus within the environment, especially in scabs or pustular material. The specifications for isolation of suspect or confirmed cases are the same as those for complete isolation, except for some modifications.

1. Private room is a must. If the patient is brought into a general hospital, personnel on the ward to which the patient is admitted should be removed to different patient care areas until proof of their successful vaccination within the past three years is obtained, or until eight days have elapsed after a successful revaccination. The patient must be placed in a private room and the door kept closed except for essential entrances and exits. (An anteroom will provide greater safety for those entering or leaving the room.)

2. Gown, gloves, mask, cap, and shoe coverings should be worn by all persons entering the room. These articles will be used only once and then discarded into an appropriate container within the room. The container will, at appropriate intervals, be double bagged and autoclaved. Its contents are sent to be incinerated, as in the case of wastes, disposable gloves, shoe coverings, and masks.

3. Linen will be double bagged and either incinerated or autoclaved (including blankets).

4. Dishes and drinking utensils are disposable. They should be double bagged and incinerated.

5. Clothing worn by the patient to the hospital and during hospitalization must be double bagged and autoclaved.

6. Letters and legal documents must be double bagged and autoclaved before they are returned to the family. They should be incinerated if not wanted by the patient.

7. Toys, jewelry, and other nonautoclavable items are to be washed with a phenolic solution and exposed to the sunlight for eight hours. Magazines, newspapers, and tissue should be double bagged and incinerated.

8. Specimens may take priority in being processed. The laboratory should be notified by telephone of any specimen that they will receive, and requested methods of handling and shipping of the specimen should be secured. Specimens must be labeled "Smallpox."

9. Visitors with previously successful vaccinations in the past three years are to be revaccinated. They may enter the contaminated room immediately after revaccination. All others may not enter until eight days after a vaccination that results in a major reaction. Persons who develop an equivocal reaction must be revaccinated. They must observe strict gown, mask, cap, glove, and shoe-covering technique.

10. Terminal disinfection requires that all furniture be wiped with phenolic disinfectant. The mattress and cover should be burned. The floor should be washed with soap and water and disinfected with formalin. The door should be closed and the window opened, exposing the room to air for 24 hours. Curtains, drapes, and other removable fabrics should be double bagged and autoclaved or incinerated.

11. Transportation is not permitted. Any emergency procedures must be done in the isolation room.

Wound and skin category

The purpose of the wound and skin category is to prevent cross infection of personnel and patients transmissible by direct wound contact or by contact with heavily contaminated articles.

COLOR CODE: PINK
SAMPLE OF WOUND AND SKIN CATEGORY DOOR CARD

VISITORS INQUIRE AT NURSES STATION BEFORE ENTERING ROOM

Gown and gloves: To be worn by all persons having direct contact with patient's linen or dressings. Discard in the room.

Masks: Use when necessary.

Hands: Everyone must wash hands well with soap and water before entering or leaving the room.

Articles: Special precautions necessary for linens, dressings, and instruments used in dressing change.

Note: _____

_____

Diseases that require use of wound and skin category

1. Abscesses and boils (any organism)
2. Conjunctivitis (newborn)
3. Gas gangrene—tetanus *(Clostridium)*
4. Staphylococcus, coagulase-positive (respiratory category precautions also used)
   a. Abscesses and boils
   b. Cellulitis
   c. Impetigo
5. Streptococcus, beta hemolytic, group A (respiratory category precautions also used)
   a. Abscesses
   b. Erysipelas
   c. Puerperal fever
6. Wound infections (any organism)
   a. Postoperative infections
   b. Posttraumatic infections
7. Venereal disease

General comments

All wounds with purulent drainage and known infection are included in this category. *Staphylococcus aureus* and beta hemolytic streptococcus are known to be infectious. However, the hazards of wound infections caused by *Proteus, Pseudomonas, Escherichia coli,* and *Clostridium perfringens* can become serious. Therefore, the same precautions are used for all.

Major precautions

Room. Private room desirable.

Gown, gloves, and mask. Gown and gloves are to be worn with all direct contact with linen or dressings. A mask is used if indicated.

Linen. Avoid vigorous movements that might spread airborne microorganisms. Double-bag all linen in isolation red bags. Use cotton blankets only. Mattresses and pillows should be well covered with plastic.

Dishes. Disposable dishes are preferred. They are placed in double plastic bag marked "Isolation" and discarded in appropriate container.

Dressings and tissues. Dressings should be handled with surgical instruments. All soiled dressings are to be sealed in double plastic bags and discarded in the soiled utility room.

Transportation. Dressing should be changed before transporting the patient, if transportation is permissible. If drainage is heavy, the nurse may place a sterile towel over the dressing. The wheelchair or cart must be washed if contaminated with drainage.

Terminal disinfection. The bed area and all areas contaminated with drainage or dressings, as well as floors, bathroom, and curtains, should be disinfected.

Visitors. Must wear gown for close patient contact and avoid contact with the patient's linen, dressings, or gown. No more than two at a time may visit.

Cultures. All cultures must be sent to the laboratory in the proper container. Place swabs in the container without contaminating the outside of the tube. If liquid pus or drainage is sent as a specimen, it should be put in a sterile tube with a screw top. The tube should be filled only half full and tightly capped. Do not contaminate the outside of the tube. If contamination occurs, the tube should be washed well before being sent to the laboratory in a clean paper bag. The outside of the bag should be marked "Isolation."

Reverse category

The purpose of the reverse category is to prevent contact of pathogenic microorganisms and uninfected persons who have seriously impaired resistance.

Diseases that signify use of reverse category

1. Agranulocytosis
2. Acute renal failure
3. Immunosuppressive therapy
4. Dermatitis (uninfected)
5. Leukemias

6. Leukopenia
7. Vaccinia with immunologic defect or immune globulin deficiency

COLOR CODE: BLUE
SAMPLE OF REVERSE CATEGORY DOOR CARD

VISITORS INQUIRE AT NURSES STATION BEFORE ENTERING ROOM

Gown and mask: To be worn by all persons entering the room. Discard *after* leaving the room.

Hands: Everyone must wash hands *well* with soap and water on entering and leaving the room.

Gloves: Worn for direct patient contact.

Articles: Linen, gowns, etc. for burn cases must be sterile when used for direct patient care.

Note: _____

_____

General comments

Patients are placed on reverse isolation only at the request of the physician. Procedures usually not associated with fatal complications, such as catheterization, may have a fatal result for this type of patient because of his low resistance to infection. It is advisable that these procedures be done only when absolutely necessary and with strict asepsis. Protection is for the patient, and only clean supplies should enter his room.

Major precautions

Room. Must be private.

Gown and mask. To be worn by all persons entering the room.

Gloves. To be worn by all who have direct patient contact.

Hands. Everyone must wash hands well with soap and water before entering or leaving the room.

Linen. All linen must be sterile for burn cases. All mattresses should be covered with plastic. The linen hamper does .1ot remain in the patient's room.

Transportation. Curtailed unless absolutely necessary. If patient is transported, he should wear a mask and gown.

Terminal disinfection. Not required.

Visitors. Must stop at the nurses station for instructions. They are limited to two at one time and must wear a gown and mask. No visitor who is known to be infected or ill may enter.

EDUCATIONAL PROGRAM

The hospital is a focal point for health care services, where community physicians and specialists concentrate their services. The total care of patients must include, directly or indirectly, the entire environment of the hospital. Since the prevention and control of infection are important elements in every phase of the hospital environment, hospitals have a common responsibility to provide prevention and control measures for the hospital population. This necessitates the training of all staff and personnel in the meaning and methods of prevention and control. It is only through concentrated and cooperative planning and effort that this training can be instituted and become a continuing process.

The professional, as well as the nonprofessional who has had little or no formal training in the fundamental concepts of microbiology, should be required to attend some type of training in the field of infection control at least once a year. The members of the professional medical and nursing staff contribute significantly to the prevention and control of infections, since their attitudes and actions set the behavior patterns for the entire hospital. By strict adherence to the rules and regulations, they may be able to instill in the nonprofessional workers a respect for proper practices at all times—not just during training or while under supervision.

The scope of the education program will depend on the individual hospital—its needs, facilities, finances, and availability of professionally trained teaching personnel. However, the content of any infection training program should be designed to share a basic knowledge of medical asepsis principles and general protective measures; to promote a healthy attitude of personnel toward the patient, his illness, and his surroundings; and to aid the worker who may have direct or indirect contact with the patient in overcoming his fear of contagion.

The educational program outlined here contains basic plans and information for various types of training sessions, as well as suggestions as to content, methods of teaching, and the addition of ingredients that will promote interest. The members of the planning committee, and especially the instructors, must have enthusiasm, ingenuity, and persistence if the hoped-for results are to be accomplished.

Instructors

Local educational resources should be explored in order to recruit the most effective instructors. Outside educational leaders may be contacted if necessary. Members of the hospital staff, such as the nurse epidemiologist, physicians, nurses, microbiologists, and department supervisors who are well versed in areas of infection control, are usually well qualified to assist with instruction or perhaps lead a training session.

To be effective an instructor should possess (1) knowledge of his subject, (2) knowledge of the inside workings of the hospital, (3) enthusiasm and interest that will inspire others, and the conviction that the job is worth doing, (4) courage to persevere against discouragement and slow acceptance, and (5) the ability to plan and organize.

Planning the program

The complexities of hospital infection control demand a broad understanding of infection control and its relation to the employees and patients. The planning committee should be chosen by the infection control committee and include the nurse epidemiologist and representatives from the education department and various other departments of the hospital. Department heads, who are not directly involved in patient-care activities, should be contacted but are not necessarily needed to actively function on the committee.

The nurse epidemiologist, because of her daily contact with personnel performance, problems, and the most recent publications, will be the most likely person to identify learning needs for the committee.

The education department has an important role in coordinating the program and in supporting the nurse epidemiologist and the infection control committee in reviewing, recommending, and developing teaching materials.

If other hospitals are to be involved, the planning committee is expanded to include selected representatives from the various hospitals. A community-wide or regional program is sponsored by several hospitals and health agencies and will require more in-depth rules. However, the basic content of the program will be similar to a general program for the individual hospital. The advantages of a cooperative program are the sharing of costs as well as the planning, and the pooling of talented instructors.

A good program should be full of inspiration, interest, information, and instruction. It should be carefully studied, well planned, and built to meet the needs and interests identified in the objectives.

The activities should provide a positive approach to the problems. It should create thinking that would result in constructive action.

Program participants

Speakers and other program participants should be asked weeks or months in advance. The date, hour, place, and length of time allotted should be clearly stated. A definite topic should be assigned, and an outline of the tentative program should be sent so that the participant will have an idea of his relationship to the program and can plan an approach to his subject.

If a panel is planned, all participants should have a few minutes together before the meeting.

Transportation, housing, and parking facilities should be arranged, and there should be a definite understanding as to traveling expenses or fees.

Arrangements for publicity should be made, introductions of guest participants should be planned.

A few days before the meeting a check should be made, if possible, with the guest speaker and other participants to be sure that all arrangements are satisfactory. Provision should be made ahead of time for tables, chairs, lighting, the microphone, drinking water, printed materials, and a test of the audio-visual equipment.

A host or hostess should be responsible to meet the guests, escort them to their proper places, and thank them properly at the end of the meeting.

The participants should be called on at the appointed time and correctly introduced. A note of appreciation should be sent, as soon as possible after the meeting, to each participant.

Introduction of speakers

Every speaker should be given a proper introduction to create a receptiveness for his remarks. The following suggestions may prove helpful in creating an attentive atmosphere:

1. Introductions should be short, courteous, and well prepared, and should include the correct name and title, the correct pronunciation of his name, and the correct title of the speech to be presented.

2. Acknowledge the presiding officer, and then the audience.

3. Use an opening sentence leading to the speaker's subject. For example, "It is a great pleasure to have with us someone who is an authority on infection control and prevention." Withhold his name until near the end of the remarks.

4. Give a few brief qualifications of the speaker and his background in the particular field of work he is presenting.

5. State the title of the speech.

6. Present him by name directly to the audience, giving full name and title—for example, "Dr. Reginald Smith, Chief of Microbiology, University Hospital."

7. Turn to the speaker and say, "Dr. Smith."

Checklist for program planners

1. Have a list of "things to do," and check it carefully and often to assure accomplishment.

2. Arrange for a printed program and an envelope of materials to be

used for reference. The envelope should contain paper, pencil, map of the area, and places to eat if meals are not provided at the meeting area.

3. Start on time.

4. Avoid long introductions.

5. Don't overcrowd the program.

6. Always provide time for questions and answers.

7. Plan the program thoroughly, anticipating unforeseen developments.

8. Plan recreation, breaks, and meals or snacks.

9. Make sure equipment is operable and in place.

10. Provide a convenient area and table for displays and handout material.

11. End the program on time.

12. Instructors should be available for at least a half hour after the close of the sessions to answer individual questions, so that time-consuming problems not specifically related to the planned program are avoided during the program itself.

Methods of presenting the program

Classes or programs on the prevention and control of infection, especially if mandatory, do not usually inspire enthusiasm in most personnel. Thoughtful planning and preparation are essential if the desired results of promoting active interest and enriching learning processes of the group are to be attained.

The principles of infection control should be presented in an effective manner that will stimulate audience participation and improve knowledge and appreciation. Methods of arousing intellectual curiosity vary with the subject, leader, audience, time involved, resources available, and creativity of the planning group. The technique must be adapted to the opportunity. Knowledge of various methods is a valuable asset to the planning committee.

Aids to the leader

1. Filmstrips
2. Slides
3. Overhead projection
4. Recordings
5. Chalkboards
6. Flannel boards
7. Charts and newsprint pads
8. Models
9. Objects (bed, oxygen tank, basin, gown, gloves, mask, etc.)

Qualifications of a leader or moderator

No matter how well prepared the initial presentation, unless the discussion is interesting, no audience will remain attentive.

In the majority of instances, the burden of creating audience interest and stimulation will rest with the leader or moderator. These leaders must be chosen with care according to the following qualifications:

1. A pleasing speaking voice
2. Sincerity, good nature, tact, and a sense of humor
3. Ability to listen, give others self-confidence, draw out the reticent, and check those who tend to monopolize
4. An intellectual honesty that allows others the right to an opinion
5. Knowledge of when to end the discussion

Methods

Lecturing, a formal presentation by an expert to a captive audience, as such, is becoming outdated in the modern concept of learning. The lecture is a valuable method of presenting material and information, but to release the intelligence of members of the audience, it should be interspersed with audiovisual aids or audience participation.

Role playing is especially helpful in a human relations situation. Members of the group, either selected or volunteer participants, will act out a life situation. There is no prepared script, since the parts are created as the role progresses. A discussion following the role playing aids in gaining an understanding of the problem presented and reaching a possible solution.

Skits are similar to role playing, except that in this type of presentation a script is prepared. Role playing and skits stress only one situation, and the time is usually limited to three minutes. This is an excellent method for communicating a key point.

The *panel* is an unrehearsed, informal method of discussion by three to six people who may sit around a table or in a semicircle and exchange views on a particular problem or issue. The discussion should flow freely, since each panel member should be knowledgeable in the subject.

At a given time, the discussion is thrown open to the audience. The well-prepared moderator may close the discussion with a short summary at a time when the audience is still deeply absorbed in the content. Whether a decision has been reached or not, it is well to end the discussion at a time that will stimulate individual thinking.

The *symposium* is similar to a panel, the difference being in the prepared-in-advance subject matter. Participants are notified well in advance and assigned a specific topic. The chairman introduces each panel member and his topic. The audience is asked to participate with questions either after each talk or at the end of the session. The chairman then summarizes the findings.

A *forum* is an outlet for free expression of the audience and is usually more lengthy than a symposium. The leader should be highly skilled in the subject and in handling audience participants. The entire meeting may consist of a talk by one selected speaker and audience questions directed to him throughout the meeting, or a panel of experts may give timed talks, after which the meeting is thrown open to the audience. The major difference between the forum and the symposium is the length of audience participation time. In the forum, as many members of the audience as possible are encouraged to air their views.

The *buzz session,* or *sectional discussion* may be either planned or extemporaneous. It is valuable for solving one particular problem, involving the entire audience in participation, or stimulating interest when the group appears restless or bored.

The leader will ask the audience to count from 1 to 6, or from 1 to 10, depending on the size of the audience. He then assigns a question or problem that may be either the same for all groups, or different for each group but related to questions or problems on the same subject in the other groups. The groups assemble according to number in various areas of the room, or in smaller rooms if they are available. After a stated length of time (6 to 10 minutes) the groups reassemble in the main room and a chairman from each group serves as a reporter to the general assembly. The leader will then summarize the reports.

Demonstration assignments are used to help evaluate the class session or to serve in the place of a written examination. The last half hour (approximate time for a group of ten) may thus be devoted to demonstrations of procedures learned.

Demonstration assignments are prepared in advance. Each member of the group draws one of the cards on which an assignment has been written, and is expected to perform the procedure written there—for example, double bagging of linen, performing handwashing technique, signing documents in isolation, emptying isolation wastebaskets, and doing exercises such as lifting, stooping, and deep breathing. (Because the double-bagging procedure will require two persons, it must be written on two separate cards.)

The instructor and the class observe as the demonstrations are carried out.

The *conference* is a 1- to 3-day program in which discussion of a subject or related subjects is led by one or more experts. Participation may vary from fifteen to hundreds, depending on the scope of the problems.

The *seminar* is a 1- to 3-day program planned for participants in a particular field under the guidance of one or more experts. The discussion-oriented program is concerned with both identifying and solving problems.

The *workshop* is a group learning process in which all types of methods of instruction may be utilized. It is planned for a specific group with a specific purpose, has a limited enrollment, meets for a definite period of time ranging from a few days to several weeks, and is often held at a university hospital or large training center.

The atmosphere of a workshop is mentally stimulating, and the participants learn by working and talking together and by drawing on each other's experience and on reference materials.

A workshop may be planned for specific groups such as nurse epidemiologists, environmental services supervisory personnel, or laboratory or nutrition supervisors, or it may serve as a rich experience for personnel of various levels who have the common goal of improving the standards of infection control in their areas.

The first session is usually devoted to getting acquainted and stating problems. The balance of the program will consist of general meetings, classroom demonstrations, lectures, discussions, clinical practices, tours, and planned study time. Recreation, breaks, and meals are necessary, since workshops usually involve the importation of concentrated knowledge in a minimum amount of time and are crowded with activities.

Experienced workshop leaders devote many months to the planning and preparing of materials so that workshop participants will grow toward a richer mental life and social satisfaction.

Many workshops carry college or certification credits. Although credits are added attractions of the workshops, they are not an essential ingredient.

At the end of the workshop, each participant is equipped with guides, materials, new skills, new attitudes, and experiences to share with the co-workers who could not attend.

A *clinic* is similar to a workshop but is based on one specific subject for participants working in the particular field. The group is usually small, since greater emphasis is placed on instruction.

Types of programs
Hospital orientation program

Because of the constant turnover of hospital personnel, an introduction to the infection control standards and the fundamental role of all personnel should be included in the hospital orientation program. Usually new employees are perplexed and insecure when they enter their new positions. This is especially true of those who have never before worked in a hospital environment. For this reason, the orientation program should be neither lengthy nor in lecture form. Overhead projection with a short narration, a filmstrip, or slides may be used in the presentation.

New interns, residents, and medical staff should become aware of the hospital infection control program as soon as possible. A *prepared packet* containing samples of the policies and admitting procedures, categories and color code, and other pertinent information should be made available.

In teaching hospitals, during the orientation of medical education students, the nurse epidemiologist may be asked to present a brief résumé of the surveillance program. At this time the packet of information may be distributed.

General program

New developments are constantly occurring in the field of infection control. The institution of new methods necessitates the training of personnel to cope with the changes. There is also a problem when personnel must become involved interdepartmentally, since infection rules will vary according to the services of the department.

Indication of needs will furnish guidelines towards planning the type of program necessary. The general program, given once a year, may consist of 1- or 2-hour briefing sessions scheduled for presentation within a controlled period of time (for example, once a week for 3 weeks), and repeated as often as necessary to allow all medical and hospital staff, personnel, and volunteers to attend. This mandatory program should have a recorded attendance in order to reimburse employees for their time and to request makeup time for those who did not attend. The general program may be expanded to an all-day session or developed, through demonstrations, lectures, or other teaching aids, to encompass a community-wide training program, especially where an interhospital infection control committee is established.

The first education program in infection control that is presented in the hospital should be a general program that briefly introduces the hospital's complete infection program. All hospital personnel do not require the same degree of instruction. For this reason the education program should be continued on a unit and departmental basis. To keep the general staff up-to-date on new developments of research, an annual briefing session should become a permanent part of the continuing education schedule. Following are the objectives:

1. To emphasize prevention as well as control
2. To utilize new developments that are appearing due to research
3. To increase the awareness of personnel to the dangers of the spread of infection

4. To develop the ability of personnel to rapidly identify signs and symptoms of infection and report them
5. To review policies and procedures and the infection program already existing

Unit and departmental teaching

Although the general program, however brief, covers the complete basic infection program of the hospital, employees should be given the opportunity to learn the skills and acquire the knowledge of prevention and control as it applies to the performance of their duties. Since training programs should be planned for the convenience of the employee, the most logical area for initiating the follow-up training is on the unit or in the department.

Unit or departmental training may be based on a particular problem that was discovered by the nurse epidemiologist or department supervisor on daily or scheduled rounds (for example, poor technique in handwashing or handling of linen), or there may be a systematic practice of transmitting information to all units and departments in a continuing process.

Established videotaped programs may be viewed through television monitors on the units or in the departments of the hospital, if the hospital is equipped for this type of program.

An inexpensive method of training small groups is through the use of the slide projector and programmed audio tape. These programs may be kept up-to-date easily by exchanging an outdated slide for a new one or by erasing the tape and re-recording.

An ideal training device is the audiovisual preparation of a complete program of infection prevention and control, including detailed procedures for nursing service and allied department personnel. Divided into specific needs, segments of this program may become a continuing process of education. For example, nursing service isolation units should view a segment on procedures pertinent to the care of the isolation patient; all units and departments should view the handwashing procedure and categories of infection; each department should routinely view the segment pertinent to that particular department; and if the nurse epidemiologist or supervisor discovers a problem on a unit or in a department, the segment relative to the problem should be viewed immediately.

The annual hospital program reinforces knowledge; the unit and departmental training programs cement it.

Educators should remain cognizant of the fact that although the audiovisual medium is a valuable training aid, it does not replace the *human element*. The learning process is stimulated when the student is able to question and receive answers.

On-the-spot teaching

All opportunities for learning must be utilized, not only in the classroom but at unexpected times. Minutes count. Sometimes a few minutes of on-the-spot teaching will prove to be of more value than a planned teaching session.

Opportunities to teach are often presented to an alert nurse epidemiologist, head nurse, department supervisor, co-worker, or physician who recognizes a possible break in the chain of infection control and applies practical knowledge through on-the-spot teaching.

Education through posters and memorandums

Posters and memorandums may be used to strengthen the educational program. Posted mottoes or reminders, in either a formal or a cartoon format, will help the hospital population form mental impressions of infection control practices.

"Wash your hands," "watch that sneeze," and "bag that dressing" may not be professional phrases, but they convey the message.

Certification of continuing education

The hospital or planning agency that sponsors an advanced program on infection control should investigate the possibility of obtaining approval from the state nurses association regarding continuing education certification for registered nurses.

Some state associations have adopted this plan of certification and have established criteria-approval committees for evaluating the tentative programs for certification.

Educational programs offered through Center for Disease Control

The Center for Disease Control (CDC) offers training and consultation for hospital staff members engaged in or selected for infection control activities. The total resource and staff of the CDC contribute to the center's training program.

Since training courses are designed to be problem specific and performance oriented, requests should be preceded by an analysis of the existing local situation. Problem definition and performance description are the two most helpful criteria to determine whether a training need exists and whether observed shortcomings can be corrected by training.

The educational services available are listed and described in CDC's *Training Bulletin,* issued for an 18-month period. The bulletin also contains information on eligibility and how to apply.*

---

*Inquiries and requests for a free copy of the *Training Bulletin* should be directed to the Center for Disease Control, Training Program, Atlanta, Ga.

Evaluation

An evaluation of any educational project is an important method of measuring the effectiveness of a program.
1. Did it achieve its objectives?
2. Did it offer worthwhile information?
3. Did it stimulate interest in infection prevention and control?
4. Did it change attitudes toward infection control?
5. Did it help to develop higher standards of surveillance?
6. Did it interpret the hospital's program of infection control?
7. How effective were the speakers? Did they convey the intended message?
8. Was there ample opportunity for audience participation?
9. Was there a cooperative spirit?
10. Was the presentation adequate to promote better job performance?
11. How can future presentations be improved?

At the close of the program an evaluation form should be given to each member of the group (see following sample). The form should be filled in and returned as soon as possible. It need not be signed.

Your honest evaluation will help us improve future programs. This form need not be signed.

TITLE OF PROGRAM: **DATE:**

1 What did you like best about this program?
2 What did you dislike about the program?
3 What speaker was the most effective?   Why?
4 Did the material presented offer new thoughts or ideas for better job performance?
5 What improvements would you suggest?
6 On the whole, how do you rate this program?

   Poor?   Fair?   Good?   Outstanding?

DATA COLLECTION, ASSIMILATION, AND INTERPRETATION

The foundation of a successful infection surveillance program is the development of a systematic reporting system. Data that are collected on a regular basis, assimilated, and analyzed may provide the means for reviewing and enforcing standards of the program of prevention or control of infections in the hospital or related institutions. It may also serve as an aid in the preparation and implementation of training programs, and as a stimulus for research. Since the usual endemic rate of infection in the hospital is known, data collection may be used to detect an increase in incidence of an infection and to determine a course of action to prevent a potential epidemic.

Methods of collecting data will depend on finances, facilities, personnel available, an interested administrator, and a working infection control committee. No program should remain static, and since no one method is all-inclusive, periodic modification is advocated.

There are three important stages in an effective reporting system: collection, assimilation, and interpretation. Each stage establishes the foundation for the next. If incomplete or inferior data are collected, assimilation and interpretation will be inaccurate, resulting in loss of time and money.

Purpose of reporting system

The purpose of the reporting system may be divided into two broad categories: specific and general. *Specific* data are sometimes necessary to gain an insight into one particular infection problem, in one or more areas where special studies may need to be performed—for example, a study of the catheterization system when a rise in urinary infections occurs; possible association of contaminated respiratory equipment with postoperative pneumonias; and intracatheter or cutdowns in association with septicemias. Each hospital has its own unique problem areas. *General* data are a prerequisite to gaining an authentic picture of infections in the total hospital environment. The data serve as a basis for the monthly infection control report to the committee.

Responsibility for collecting data

Once a decision has been made as to the purpose of the data, the next step is the delegation of a responsible individual to perform the duties of collection. The most appropriate individual is the *nurse epidemiologist,* who is trained in patient care and whose experience and interest in the principles of epidemiology are supported by a fundamental knowledge of biostatistics. It is essential that the nurse epidemiologist and the chairman of the infection control committee have a good working relationship.

Even a full-time nurse epidemiologist cannot accomplish the task of surveillance without assistance. Personnel in all departments should be alert to infection problems and methods of prevention, and should report on a current and systematic basis to the nurse epidemiologist. Reports such as culture results on formula, ice machines, and environmental cleanliness; personnel health involvement; and charge nurse checks on infection diagnoses or developments will reflect the workability of the surveillance program. A close association with the utilization of the microbiology laboratory is essential to a properly functioning program.

Methods of collection, assimilation, and interpretation

Some hospitals rely entirely on a sampling of infections for their surveillance program. Although decisions may evolve from sampling, there is always some uncertainty attached to it.

The use of computers has become a common method of assimilation and interpretation. The correct information must be carefully collected before it can be accurately fed into the computer. See Figs. 3-9 and 3-10.

Cut-off time will depend on the purpose and scope of the data collection. A choice reporting system is the daily accumulative collection of statistical data on a monthly and yearly basis, in which both community- and hospital-associated infections are classified by type, duration, and spread as it affects the hospital.

The reporting system described here may be easily adapted to the needs of most hospitals. The process of data collection is basically the same for both specific and general purposes; only the scope will be expanded.

Planning for a systematic gathering of data should include consideration of sources that may indicate infections; areas in the hospital where data may be found; tools that may be used in collecting the data; and some method of coding the information.

Indications of infection on patient's chart or departmental reports

1. Diagnosis
   a. Known infections such as hepatitis or measles
   b. Suspicion of infection, caused by fever of undetermined origin (FUO) and diarrhea

SURVEY ON URINARY INFECTIONS		Date_____ To_____			
Name of the Patient and Hospital Number	Date of Admittance	Date – Time Catheterized	Foley Inserted Date--Time	Foley Removed Date -- Time	Irrigate Yes - - No

Fig. 3-9. Form for survey of urinary infections illustrates *specific* purpose of data collections.

2. Urine reports (urinalysis)
3. Chemistry reports (serum glutamic oxaloacetic transaminase (SGOT), complete blood count [CBC], etc.)
4. Culture reports (sputum, blood, urine, wound exudate, spinal fluid, etc.)
5. Temperature sheets (sudden change in temperature)
6. Medicine sheets (antibiotics prescribed)
7. X-ray reports (respiratory, gastrointestinal, etc.)
8. Physician's orders (order for *stat* cultures or medicines)
9. Patient's care plan and treatment sheet ("hot wet packs" or "soaks")
10. Specific problems (diarrhea in personnel, cloudy I.V. solution)

Current Month * Last Month ** Month:_____			INFECTION CONTROL REPORT																	Please Read & Destroy
COMMUNITY – ASSOCIATED			HOSPITAL–ASSOCIATED (NOSOCOMIAL)																		REMARKS
TYPE	*	**	Unit / Ward	Discharges		Respiratory		Urine		Wound & Skin		G. I.		Other		Total					
				*	**	*	**	*	**	*	**	*	**	*	**	*	%	**	%		
Respiratory			Medical Ward 1																		
Urine			2																		
Gastro–Intestinal			3																		
Wound & Skin			4																		
Other			5																		
Viral Exanthem			6																		
			7																		
Meningitis			8																		
Encephalitis			Total Medical																		
Hepatitis			Surgical A																		
T.B.			B																		
Mumps			C																		
			D																		
			Total Surgical																		
			Pediatrics																		
			OB/GYN																		
Total			NURSERY																		
NOSOCOMIAL OTHERS			Total																		
(List)			Culture: E. Coli																		
			Pseudo.																		
			Proteus																		
			Enter.																		
			K. Pneu.																		
Total			H. Influ.																		
ADMISSION			Staph +																		
DISCHARGE			Strep fec.																		
% NOSOCOMIAL			B.H. Strep not A B.H. Strep "A"																		
% PATIENTS ADMITTED WITH INFECTION			Other Gr. – Other Gr. +																		
			Total																		

Fig. 3-10. Monthly infection control report form illustrates *general* purpose of data collection.

11. Incident report of infection (form to be filled in by nurse or physician)
12. Nurse-physician consultation (oral or written)
13. Environmental report (monthly on special areas)
14. Nursery formula report (weekly)

Sources of data

1. Admitting department
2. Laboratory
3. X-ray department
4. Ward rounds
5. Medical records department (discharge charts)

Tools for collecting data

1. Hospital census sheet (daily record of all in-patients)
2. Hospital admission report (daily record of all admissions)
3. Patient's chart (current composite record of patient's hospital stay)
4. Hospital discharge report (daily record of all patients who were discharged the previous day)

Coding of information

A coding system should be individually devised to tabulate the daily collection.

$$\text{Example:} \quad \begin{array}{ll} \text{U} & \text{Urinary} \\ \text{Wd} & \text{Wound} \\ \text{Resp} & \text{Respiratory} \\ \text{GI} & \text{Gastrointestinal} \end{array}$$

Colors may be used to identify areas or to signify tabulation. For example; *green* may be used to indicate that the patient's chart has not been checked but that the patient had a suspicious or known infection on admission, or on the laboratory report or x-ray report. *Black* may be used to indicate that the patient's chart was reviewed "today" and not yet tabulated, and *red* may indicate that tabulation on the accumulative work sheet has been accomplished. A *black* line through a name on the daily census sheet may indicate that the patient's chart was reviewed and no infection was noted.

The word *yes* could be used to indicate a hospital-associated infection, and *no* to indicate a community-associated infection.

Daily data collection

1. *Admitting department.* The daily admission sheet may be quickly scanned for the diagnosis of each patient. If a known or suspicious indi-

cation is found, the patient's name may be circled in green on the daily census sheet, to be checked later.

2. *Laboratory.* Urine, chemistry, and culture reports are checked. If the culture shows many pathogens, the patient's name may be circled in green on the daily census sheet. In many cases the pathologist has already reported his findings to the physician. If cultures that are incubating in the laboratory at 8 A.M. are immediately reported to the physician, the patient may be in isolation by noon. Postmortem reports are also reviewed in the laboratory.

3. *X-ray department.* If statements pertaining to respiratory or gastrointestinal infections or abscesses are found on x-ray reports, the patient's name may be circled in green as a further check.

4. *Ward rounds.* The patient's chart is carefully reviewed for clues to possible developing infections: temperature sheets, cardex, culture orders, treatments, antibiotics, or other indications. A talk with the charge nurse may reveal such problems as suspicious wounds not cultured, which should be immediately brought to the attention of the physician responsible for infection control in that area.

After the patient's chart has been checked thoroughly, any infections found are charted in black on the daily census sheet as community or hospital associated.

If a hospital-associated infection is suspected, and the physician has made no indication on the chart, an incident report of infection (Fig. 3-11) is filled in and placed on the patient's chart for the physician to note confirmation or denial of infection present, and the nurse epidemiologist is notified.

This report is not a permanent part of the patient's chart but is sent to the nurse epidemiologist when the patient is discharged. The infection is noted on the census sheet.

In addition to the incident report of infection, a nosocomial case card (Fig. 3-12) is filled out by the nurse epidemiologist and kept by her for the monthly report.

5. *Daily discharge sheet.* Patient's charts that were not previously reviewed on ward rounds are checked in the medical records department after the patient is discharged. If a nosocomial infection is discovered, with no indication by the physician on the chart, the incident report of infection is filled in and filed in medical records for the physician's signature. The nosocomial case card is also filled out and retained by the nurse epidemiologist. All infections discovered on the discharge charts are coded on the discharge sheet.

6. *Incident report of infection.* Some hospitals require an incident report of infection on all infections, both community and hospital associated.

However, this requires that extra time be spent by the charge nurse, nurse epidemiologist, or physician. For this reason, incident reports of infection should probably be used only for a known or suspected nosocomial infection not previously noted on the chart by the physician. It is a recognized method of obtaining confirmation of the infection as a nosocomial type.

INCIDENT REPORT OF INFECTIONS THIS FORM MAY ORIGINATE WITH THE PERSON SUSPECTING AN INFECTION: I. On admission of patient having infection. 2. At the time an infection appears during hospital stay.	STENCIL CLEARLY

DATE OF THIS REPORT: _____ DATE OF ADMISSION: _____

DIAGNOSIS:_____

NATURE OF INFECTION:_____

DATE OF SURGERY: _____ O.R. ROOM NO: _____ TIME OF SURGERY:_____

TYPE OF SURGERY: _____

_____

NURSE or CLERK

TO BE COMPLETED BY PHYSICIAN

DOES THIS PATIENT HAVE AN INFECTION ACQUIRED SINCE ADMISSION: [ ] YES [ ] NO

NATURE OF INFECTION: _____

APPARENT SOURCE:_____

_____

ATTENDING PHYSICIAN

LABORATORY INVESTIGATION

CULTURE DONE: [ ] YES [ ] NO

SOURCE OF CULTURE: _____

ORGANISM ISOLATED: _____

_____

INFECTION CONTROL NURSE

THIS FORM IS NOT A PART OF THE PERMANENT MEDICAL RECORD

Fig. 3-11. Incident report of infection.

Name:				NOSOCOMIAL CASE CARD					
Month	Adm.	Disc.	Hosp. No.	Age	Room	Physician	Surgeon	Isolation	
								Yes No	

Diagnosis:		Type		Organism	Antibiotic		S	R
		GI		Bacteroides	Ampicillin			
Surgery:		Resp		B.H. Str. A	Bacitracin			
		Urine		B.H. Not A	Carbenicillin			
No. Hours:	Room No.: Date:	Wound		Diphtheroid	Cephalothin			
		Other		E. Coli	Chloramphenicol			
Remarks:	Underlying Process:	Predisposing Factors:		Enterobact.	Colistin			
				K. Pneu.	Erythromycin			
	CA	Cutdown		H. Inf.	Garamycin			
	Diabetic	Drains		Proteus	Kanamycin			
	Renal Dis.	Dressings		Pseudomonas	Lincomycin			
	Paralysis	Equipment		Salmonella	Methicillin			
	Burn	Foley		Serratia	Naldixic Acid			
	Coma	GU Inst.		Shigilla	Nitrofurantoin			
	Decubitus	Intracath		Staph +	Nystatin			
	Steroids	IV		Staph −	Penicillin			
	Radiation	Trach		Strep Fec.	Streptomycin			
				Other Gr. +	Sulfa			
				Other Gr. −	Tetracycline			

Fig. 3-12. Nosocomial case card.

7. *Physician's office.* Physicians should notify the nurse epidemiologist or infection control departmental officer of any infections that develop after discharge from the hospital. However, if the nurse epidemiologist discovers indications of a developing infection when the patient's chart is checked on discharge, a follow-up call to the physician's office may be in order.

Tabulating

All information collected is recorded in the appropriate places. An accumulative work sheet for community-associated infections is convenient (Fig. 3-13).

The nosocomial case cards are placed in a current file to be used later for the monthly report.

Black code marks from the daily census and daily discharge sheets should be transferred in red to the new daily sheets the following morning, in preparation for fresh data collection.

Assimilation of data

Monthly report to the infection control committee (Fig. 3-10).

Information for the monthly report is derived from the work sheet (Fig. 3-13) and the nosocomial case card (Fig. 3-12).

WORK SHEET				
COMMUNITY-ASSOCIATED OR NON-ACQUIRED INFECTIONS MONTH _____				
TYPES G I	RESPIRATORY	URINE	WOUND & SKIN	OTHERS

AMEBIOSIS
DIARRHEA
SALMONELLA
SHIGELLA
STOOLS
	ASTHMA
	BRONCHITIS
	CROUP
	FLU
	PNEUMONIA
	SPUTUM
	TRACH
			ABSCESS
			EAR
			EYE
				<u>DISEASES OF INFECTION</u>
				CHICKEN POX
				HEPATITIS:
				    Serum
				    Infectious
				HERPES ZOSTER
				MENINGITIS
				MONONUCLEOSIS
				MUMPS
				SEPTICEMIA
				TUBERCULOSIS
				VIRAL EXANTHEM
				    Measles
				    Scarlet fever
				
				<u>SITES</u>
				BLOOD
				CATH TIP (IV CVP)
				CORD (Umbilical NB)
				IV FILTER
				SPINAL FLUID
				VAG (lochia, PID)

Fig. 3-13. Community-associated infection monthly work sheet.

Figures from the previous month's report are included for comparison of data. Discharges by unit and service are necessary if rates of unit and service infections are required.

Since nosocomial case cards may be permanently filed alphabetically, the nurse epidemiologist may prefer to list nosocomial cases of the current report for quick reference (Fig. 3-14). Only one copy is necessary and may be filed with the original of the monthly report.

All nosocomial case cards of current patients should be kept in an active file until the patient is discharged; a notation of the infection is carried in red on future census sheets. However, the infection is not listed on future monthly reports unless an additional infection develops.

The total number of admissions for the current month and the total number of monthly discharges by unit and service are usually obtained from the medical records department. The number of patients with infec-

Discharge Data	WARD	Patients' Name	Type	Surgery	Culture

LIST OF NOSOCOMIALS   Month _____

Fig. 3-14. List of nosocomial (hospital-associated) infections—monthly work sheet.

tions that were cultured during the month may be obtained from the laboratory.

Interpretation

Effective surveillance consists not only in the collection of data but also in its interpretation. During the daily accumulation, evidences of cross infections or infections from a common source are investigated immediately. They are also reflected in the monthly report.

Rates of infection by site, service, unit, or pathogen may be calculated according to the individual needs of the hospital.

Statistics are only as good as the use made of them. The data report must accurately convey the specific items intended.

The completed monthly report is reviewed by the infection control committee, and after approval by the committee, copies should be given to the appropriate persons involved, such as the hospital administrator and the head nurse of each unit, to keep them informed of the progress of the hospital infection control program.

Problem solving

A sudden or progressive rise in any hospital-associated infection should alert the surveillance officer to the necessity of an immediate investigation of the cause, such as contaminated food, contaminated surgical instruments, person-to-person spread, or a possible epidemic.

Investigating a hospital-associated epidemic

Epidemic investigation relies almost entirely on fact gathering. The bacteriology laboratory is the best possible source available for confirming the diagnosis of an epidemic.

Once the diagnosis has been confirmed and the total number of cases determined, the investigation will demand the full attention of the infection control committee and the nurse epidemiologist (surveillance officer).

The investigative program should consider all unusual situations. Expert consultation may be required to aid in analyzing data collected if the source is difficult to identify.

The attack rate, a figure that reflects the number of cases under investigation in proportion to the total number of individuals involved in the risk, will demonstrate the number of people who acquired the disease and the number of exposed persons who did not acquire the disease. For example:

$$\text{Attack rate} = \frac{\text{Number of new infections}}{\text{Number of patients in hospital}} \times 100 \text{ (expressed in \%)}$$

After all pertinent evidence has been analyzed and the source established, measures are taken for controlling the present epidemic and for preventing future occurrences.

An excellent source of community epidemic prevention and rapid identification is through the inter hospital infection control committee. Since members of this group meet monthly and discuss hospital infection problems, they are aware of any increase in incidence or of the occurrence of an unusual infection.

An effective surveillance program and an alert nurse epidemiologist or surveillance officer are still the best resources in the prevention and control of hospital-associated epidemics.

Handling a nursery outbreak

Since nurseries are high-risk areas, a detailed program of action for a nursery diarrhea outbreak may be of value in establishing nursery policies and procedures.

The following procedure is based on a hypothetical instance in which five babies acquired explosive diarrhea in one day in the same nursery. The nursery charge nurse may become aware of a possible epidemic or communicable problem either through a physician who is attending one of the babies or through the laboratory.

Program of action

1. The charge nurse should immediately notify the following:
   a. Nurse epidemiologist

    b. Infection control chairman or Pediatrics infection control officer

    c. Physicians of all infants in the contaminated nursery

  2. She should then request that stool specimens be sent immediately to the laboratory for culture and determination of pathogen sensitivity.

  3. The contaminated nursery must be closed to further admissions and all babies with diarrhea placed in a separate nursery. The technique established for the enteric category should be immediately instituted. The exposed babies remaining in the contaminated nursery should be carefully observed for any signs of diarrhea. Babies in both areas should not be taken from the nursery. Mothers may breast-feed babies in a special room in the nursery section.

  4. Physicians should authorize cultures of stool specimens of all mothers of the babies who contracted diarrhea.

  5. A possible break in aseptic techniques, especially in handwashing, should be investigated.

  6. If it becomes necessary to investigate further, all personnel, including physicians and students who had contact with the infants two days prior to the outbreak, should have stool specimens cultured.

  7. Results of the stool cultures should be carefully analyzed. If the source is still elusive, formula, water, and perhaps nasal secretions of attending personnel should be cultured.

  8. If the source proves to be a mother or her baby, they should be treated, and then on discharge the problem will be solved. If personnel are the source of contamination, they should not be allowed in the nursery area until three stool cultures prove negative.

  9. When all infants involved in the outbreak are discharged, both contaminated nurseries are terminally cleaned and cultured.

  10. The nurse epidemiologist then prepares a confidential report of the entire proceedings for the infection control committee chairman.

  In complicated cases, outside help may be obtained from the public health department or the Center for Disease Control, Atlanta.

Reportable diseases

  A working relationship between the hospital and the public health department is vital to rapid identification of an epidemic problem in the community. All communicable diseases must be reported to the public health authorities, and epidemics may be prevented if prompt notification is received by the health department. Because it is the responsibility of the physician to report these diseases to the health department, he should have up-to-date knowledge of reportable diseases and the reporting methods.

  Each state designates the reportable diseases they feel should be kept under strict surveillance; a list of these diseases and the method of notification may be obtained from the state health department.

Most states use a small printed card for reporting communicable diseases to the health department. It is signed by the physician and contains the patient's name, address, age, and sex, the diagnosis, the date of the report, and any other pertinent information.

Following is a general list of reportable diseases:

Amebiasis
Brucellosis
Chickenpox
Coccidioidomycosis
Diarrhea (cause undetermined)
German measles
Hepatitis, infectious
Histoplasmosis
Influenza
Leptospirosis
Malaria
Measles (rubeola)
Mononucleosis, infectious
Mumps
Psittacosis
Q fever
Respiratory diseases, acute
    (cause undetermined)

Ringworm (scalp)
Salmonella infection
    Typhoid
    Paratyphoid
    Other
Shigellosis
Staphyloccocal infection
Streptoccocal infection, grade A
    Rheumatic fever
    Scarlet fever
    Other
Tetanus
Trachoma
Tularemia
Whooping cough (pertussis)

Diseases to be reported immediately on confidential morbidity card:

Tuberculosis—all forms
Venereal diseases
Anthrax
Botulism
Diphtheria
Encephalitis, arthropod-borne
Hepatitis, serum

Leprosy
Meningitis, meningococcal
Plague
Poliomyelitis
Rabies in man
Smallpox
Typhus (specify)

CHAPTER FOUR

Meeting the emotional needs of the isolation patient

Individuals differ in the degree and intensity of emotional behavior during illness. Even under normal circumstances, the emotional element requires consideration, but the best-adjusted patient will become apprehensive at the thought of being isolated. If the first hospitalization experience necessitates isolation, the traumatic overtones may assume gigantic proportions. The sudden change in routine, the strangeness of surroundings, and the limited activities, resulting from the strict rules and regulations of isolation, may create emotional difficulties for the patient that prove greater than the illness for which he is being treated. Emotional trauma may, in the extreme, actually result in the death of the patient.

Patients have various responses to isolation, such as apprehension, anxiety, and frequently, guilt. These responses may take the overt form of abusive, resentful, aggressive, and, at times, withdrawal behavior. Anger is not only an expression of the patient's frustrations but often becomes an outlet for the frustrations felt by his family. It serves as a camouflage for desperately frightened individuals whose fears of contagion often override their desire to be with the patient.

The nurse who is sensitive to individual variations in stress situations may ease the pressures of isolation for the patient and his family by providing emotional support, education, and interpretation of isolation.

No patient should remain in isolation without some basic understanding of what he may expect. If, on admission, the patient is exceedingly ill or the family emotionally upset, they should not be burdened with details. When they are capable of receiving and assimilating such information, a thorough presentation of the procedures of isolation and of the transmission modes of the infection, as well as a rationale for the strict protective precautions that must be taken, may be offered.

What may seem to be a simple routine isolation procedure to the hospital staff is alien to the average patient, and his methods of defending himself against anxiety and the unknown may cause him to be uncooperative. Optimum results may be achieved when the patient understands how significant cooperation is to his recovery.

The excessive washing of hands, gowning, masking, and gloving implies to the anxious patient that he is being rejected. Hospitals in Tucson, Arizona, have adopted the phrase "protective care" to replace the word "isolation," thus emphasizing the care being offered rather than the state of being alone or rejected. The results have been positive.

The excessive demands of the patient in isolation may become extremely frustrating to the nurse. For example, he may invent excuses to bring her into the room and keep her there as long as possible. However, the patient is lonely, and the nurse may help to alleviate his loneliness by visiting him whenever possible and by developing some recreational or diversional therapeutic activities. Incoming and outgoing telephone calls and mail help the patient to feel less isolated; flowers bring warmth and beauty to the room; television and radio may fill some of his empty time and be a source of enjoyment.

In some cases the infection problem is less severe, so that indirect care may not require a gown or mask. A nurse or visitor may reduce the patient's feeling of isolation by sitting nearby and allowing him to express his thoughts.

Some hospitals have isolation areas that are separated within a room, thereby allowing visitors or staff to communicate with the patient without the necessity of entering the protected area.

Religious faith is comforting to many persons, particularly in a time of illness. The clergy are encouraged to visit regularly if their services are requested by the patient.

PEDIATRIC PATIENT IN ISOLATION

The new experience of isolation is threatening to the apprehensive child because emotional development is incomplete. Children require more reassurance since they have difficulty grasping the reasons for isolation. Explanations may help reduce anxiety, but a great number of repetitions will probably be necessary. Removal from familiar home surroundings to a strange place results in insecurity. Most children are active and forgetful, and their attention span is short. Dull rules and procedures that emphasize negatives and restrict physical activity seem unfair and suspicious, and they thus promote rebellion, particularly in a situation that is already threatening. Adults may find an outlet by complaining about their food or the service, but children vent their feelings by crying, withdrawing, or rebelling.

Making a game of the rules, keeping the child busy with things that interest him, establishing a bedtime routine similar to his accustomed home situation, allowing him a favorite toy and blanket, and encouraging him to pursue hobbies, read, work puzzles, or watch TV will divert his attention for a time. However, any materials used in isolation must be those which may either be burned or properly disinfected later.

The very young child is more demanding than most older children, since his fears and needs are concentrated on love and security. Parents may offer the greatest emotional support to the isolated child of any age, but their presence is of great assistance to the needs of the infant.

Not every nurse is geared to work with children. Nursing personnel for pediatric isolation areas should be especially selected for their patience and ability to adequately handle the specific problems of children and their parents, and to receive training in the special procedures required in these areas. Although isolation procedures are taught to children, preferably as a game, the great responsibility in prevention and control must be borne by the nurse and/or parents. It is imperative that parents realize the importance of the role they will play while their child is in this area of the hospital, and that they understand the procedures clearly in order to cooperate fully.

TEEN-AGER IN ISOLATION

Probably the most difficult isolation patient will be the teen-ager. The adult accepts the inevitable, love will suffice for the young child, but the teen-ager feels abandoned. In addition to his frustrations, he refuses to accept any rational explanation as to why this catastrophe should happen to him. Consequently, his responses are associated with a sense of inferiority and may surface in such a rebellious and demanding nature as to completely disrupt routine in the isolation area. It is essential that the staff avoid displaying their irritation and concentrate efforts on establishing rapport with the patient.

His ego needs to be satisfied, and if this goal cannot be accomplished in a positive manner, he will use a negative approach for effect. The fact that friends must follow rules if they are to be permitted visitation privileges sometimes promotes a satisfying sense of importance—he feels that he is worth the effort. Special attention to his moods and temperament may result in opportunities to forestall temper tantrums. Conversation should be encouraged by a nurse who is a good listener. His opinions on ways of improving isolation activities for his age group may be well worth hearing.

Sympathetic understanding is still the fundamental factor in coping with most of his isolation problems.

FAMILY

An interpretation to the family regarding the disease of the patient, the reasons for isolation, and the family's role in helping the patient and in the prevention and control of disease will ease many of the confusions and frustrations that family members are certain to have. An open discussion of contagion and of the manner in which the family may visit the patient and still be free of contagion will relieve their fears and encourage intelligent visiting.

DISSEMINATING INFORMATION

There are a number of ways to disseminate information regarding procedures and precautions during isolation. Verbal instructions at the nurses station, even if they seem repetitive, are always worthwhile because they more nearly guarantee a proper interpretation of the rules than any other method. Coupled with verbal instructions are written materials. The most effective method is the specific use of door cards and brochures.

Door cards explain in writing the type of infection encountered and the precautions to be taken in a specific instance, and they are designed for the use of personnel and visitors rather than the patient. They provide a good method for the review of important facts at each visit to a given isolation patient.

A brochure, which covers the general subject of isolation, the precautions taken, and reasons for them, includes information for patient, family, and visitor. The style and format may range from comic to serious, but the brochure should not be written too technically because the audience will include persons unschooled and totally uninformed in infection control as well as the broadly educated and well informed, and it must communicate its message to both.

The best-received brochures seem to be those which liberally use interesting, pertinent illustrations to supplement and accent the written material.

A brochure should include the following information:

1. *General remarks* will present the meaning of isolation and an explanation as to why isolation is necessary; the types of protective care given; a discussion of the fact that special rules and procedures must be observed; and the concept that protective care is not only for the patient but for the visitor as well.

2. The *patient* receives an explanation of procedures required of him; the rules that will affect his meals, mail, clothing, and other articles; a statement of the rules of visitation; and encouragement to question the nurse when in doubt about any rule or procedure.

3. The *visitor* receives a brief explanation of protective care; advice to report to the nurses station before visiting; and a discussion of general procedures required of visitors and the rules that must be followed.

It is important to emphasize in all media of communication that the purpose of isolating the patient has a positive rather than a negative basis.

CHAPTER FIVE
Legal aspects of
hospital-associated infections

The possibility of legal involvement is not the major factor in the prevention and control of infections in the hospital. However, court case records establish the fact that litigations are brought against hospitals when hospital-associated infections develop, and that lawsuits involving hospital-associated infections are on the increase. Although negligence in infectious cases is difficult to prove, the very fact that legal action is taken reflects on the standards of care in the institution and places the health facility and its infection control system on trial.

Patients have a right to expect the hospital environment to be as germ free as possible, but it is also understood that the hospital, because of its very reason for existence, cannot be completely free of infection. Infection enters the hospital environment in several ways: through the infected patient, the visitor, the personnel, and food and pests. The hospital has limited control over visitors, patients, or personnel who introduce unrecognized infections into its facility. Although hospitals are required to use reasonable care in controlling the spread of existing infection and in preventing new infections, they do not guarantee that there will be no infection. The hospital has no specific duty to warn patients that they might acquire a hospital-associated infection. Theoretically, the public is aware that the hospital is expected to care for all types of diseases and that the individual may enter the hospital for the express reason that he does have a disease. Nevertheless, the fact that hospitals do have infections will naturally create certain legal problems.

Liability suits for hospital-associated infections may be based on the law of torts, the doctrine of *res ipsa loquitur,* or the doctrine of *respondeat superior.*

A *tort* (Latin *tortus,* "to twist") is a legal wrong, either intentional or unintentional, committed by one person against the person or property of another. To compensate for such a private legal wrong, the law permits the harmed person to bring a civil action against the wrongdoer to recover a sum of money. Merely contracting an infection in the hospital is not in itself evidence of negligence on the part of the hospital. The patient must produce evidence of hospital negligence and that such negligence resulted in the infection.

Res ipsa loquitur ("the thing speaks for itself") is a doctrine that applies in situations where the infection would not ordinarily occur if those in exclusive control had used proper care. In this case, the hospital must prove that it did not commit the act.

Respondeat superior ("let the master respond") is a legal doctrine that creates liability on the part of the employer for those negligent acts of his employees which were committed within the scope of their employment. Medical staff members are seldom considered hospital employees because they are independent contractors who receive compensation from the patient and not the hospital. However, interns and residents are considered employees because they perform their duties under the supervision of hospital staff physicians.

Charitable immunity is a rule that nonprofit hospitals cannot be held liable for the negligence of their employees. However, few states still accept this immunity.

Governmental immunity is a rule which states that a governmental body cannot be sued for the negligent acts of its employees without its consent. There are certain limitations in the Federal Tort Act that now make it possible to bring suit against the federal government to recover for negligent injuries caused by its employees.

Frequent reevaluation of the established hospital standards of care is necessary, since courts take into consideration whether the hospital exercised a reasonable standard of care to avoid infection, or whether the infection was caused by a specific act.

Functioning according to community standards is no longer a good defense against liability since national standards have been established. State agencies that have jurisdiction over the licensing of hospitals have established necessary rules and regulations governing the operation of hospitals, and included in these rules are standards that relate to infection control. However, high standards alone do not insulate a hospital against liability, especially in high-risk situations where a maximum degree of care is demanded. A hospital may follow national standards and still be subjected to liability.

Since there is no assured way to completely avoid liability for nosocomial infections, the hospital must build a stronger defense against infection and any possible break in the chain of control. A review of circumstances that have led to court actions involving hospital-associated infections may aid in reevaluating existing situations in local hospitals and may thus minimize the occurrence of litigation. The following circumstances may prove to be a basis for legal action:

1. Cross infection due to nurses' negligence in failing to wash their hands between patients; unkempt attire of personnel
2. Inadequate ventilation and methods of waste disposal; defective hospital or medical equipment
3. Improper sterilization or failure to sterilize operating or injecting instruments; unsterile manual examinations; use of unsterile hypodermic needles for injections; improper care of wounds
4. Deviations from standards set for cleaning floors, walls, or isolation rooms
5. "Clean" operations performed in the same operating room immediately following a "dirty" operation
6. Negligence in not calling a superior when a problem arises that might lead to infection and that requires immediate care
7. Allowing hospital personnel to work without preemployment examinations or placing personnel in high-risk areas without proper precautions, such as nose or stool cultures
8. Failure to maintain standards of care when sterility is required throughout a procedure
9. Failure to administer antibody therapy when an infection occurs (merely cleaning the site with an antiseptic)
10. Failure to make isolation facilities available for patients with a communicable disease; causing unnecessary exposure by failure to isolate a patient with a suspected infection until the infection is proved
11. Failure to perform duties according to standards prevailing for a particular type of infection
12. Committing or omitting an act contrary to infection policies set up by the Joint Commission of Accreditation or the state licensure
13. Using blood for transfusions that has not been properly checked for hepatitis (some states regard blood transfusion as a sale, whereas others regard it as a service; however, suits have resulted in both cases)

Detailed facts and court cases have been quoted in bulletins from the Center for Disease Control and are available on request.

A good defense against legal redress is to take all possible precautions; schedule regular inspections of the hospital by experienced maintenance men, especially the air conditioning equipment; keep adequate records; and maintain contact with the patient after discharge by follow-up through the physician's office.

The infection control committee will benefit by keeping abreast of new legislation. For example, an Arizona statute states that records and minutes of the infection control committee are immune to subpoena if the community has a medicolegal committee (Arizona revised statute 36-445, Arizona legislature, 1971).

The use of the term "hospital-acquired infection" might serve as a basis for suit because it states, in fact, that the infection was acquired in the hospital. Since there are gradations of nosocomial infections, perhaps a more acceptable term, such as "hospital-associated infection," might be used.

Even the best safeguards are not enough, but infections pose a problem which physicians, hospital administrations, and responsible health officials recognize. They are combining their efforts to find methods for prevention and control.

CHAPTER SIX

Interaction of health services and the hospital infection program

Health agencies share a major goal of the hospital—to protect the public from disease. In many localities the hospital is the focal point for community health services, but too often, even in these localities, interaction between the hospitals and the outside agencies and services available to the patient is not fully realized.

Through a sharing of ideas and research, as well as cooperation in the implementing of community prevention and control programs, the mutual goal may be realized and maintained.

AMERICAN HOSPITAL ASSOCIATION (AHA)

The American Hospital Association's Committee on Infections Within the Hospital provides standards for nosocomial infection control. A handbook, *Infection Control in the Hospital,* has been compiled by the American Hospital Association and contains information pertinent to effective control. This association is available as a resource in any hospital-associated problems.

CENTER FOR DISEASE CONTROL (CDC)

The Center for Disease Control is part of the Health Services and Mental Health Administration, which, in turn, is one of the three major divisions of the Public Health Service, United States Department of Health, Education, and Welfare. It has the distinction of being one of the few major components of the Public Health Service with headquarters outside the Washington, D. C., area.

CDC has been located in Atlanta, Georgia, since the organization began as the Office of Malaria Control in War Areas (MCWA) in 1942. At the end of the war the MCWA began a laboratory training program on the diagnosis of parasitic infections, to assist in maintaining the health of returning servicemen.

In 1946 the Surgeon General, recognizing the broad base of competence in the control of a number of infectious diseases that had developed in MCWA, directed that the name be changed to Communicable Disease Center. In 1970 the name was changed again to Center for Disease Control, since its activities encompass other preventable diseases also.

The mission of the CDC is to carry out a program of applied research and training in the prevention and control of preventable diseases, to provide epidemic aid, to administer the Foreign Quarantine Program of the Public Health Service, and to provide consultation and other assistance to the states in their effort to prevent and contral infectious disease.

The Hospital Infections Section carries out a variety of projects in the epidemiology and control of hospital infections. The services listed below are only a few of those available.

1. To develop and evaluate surveillance systems
2. To provide epidemic aid to hospitals on request through state departments of health
3. To provide diagnostic services to states on specimens that require specialized testing
4. To study disinfection and sterilization of hospital equipment
5. To offer consultation and technical assistance

The Training Program, in close cooperation with the Hospital Infections Section, plans, develops, and presents educational activities in hospital infections control and prevention as part of its mission.

PUBLIC HEALTH SERVICE (PHS)

The United States Health Service is concerned with the prevention and control of diseases, and with the protection of the public, on a local, state, and national level.

A vital contribution to the hospital's program of prevention and control of infections is made by the health facilities environmentalist, who works on a local level with hospitals and environments that affect health.

Many hospitals employ a hospital sanitarian, whose position as a key member of the patient care team is (1) to service all areas of the hospital environment for the purpose of preventing the spread of disease-producing organisms and (2) to coordinate the hospital with the public health office.

The services of the public health environmentalist are free to health facilities, and his duties will vary in the individual states. Basically the environmentalist may be compared to an auditor who finds evidence of impending deficiencies and brings it to the attention of the person with the appropriate area of responsibility. Unfortunately, in many institutions the environmentalist is considered to be a detective who threatens administrative control.

The environmentalist may be of inestimable value to hospitals by serving in an advisory capacity—for example, recommending a hospital sanitation program and assisting in setting up and maintaining the program. The hospital profits by having a specialist familiar with problems yet far enough removed to be able to recognize a change in the picture that may be overlooked by a person who is too closely involved.

Since no facility can be perfect in all respects, recommendations of the environmentalist prepares the hospital for state inspection and for reports that must be made to government agencies. The environmentalist does not expect great improvements to be accomplished overnight. However, follow-up of recommendations is necessary after a reasonable time lapse.

Infection control duties of the environmentalist include the following:
1. General licensing inspection of the physical plant: walls, ceilings, floors, ventilation systems, and mechanical and electrical equipment
2. Sanitation inspection: dietary service, water facilities, handwashing facilities on units, private wells, ice (storage and distribution procedures), and a monthly bacteriologic sampling of these areas; disposal of sewage and waste
3. Housekeeping, including cleaning procedures (checking of detergents, disinfectants, and cleaning equipment for best results), and linen storage and handling
4. Therapy pool: inspection and sampling of water
5. Bacterial surveillance program includes a check on all cultures taken for the environmental service

The environmentalist's job is strictly with conditions of environmental health and does not include patient care procedures.

For any problem or study requiring specialized help, the infection control committee may contact the Public Health Service, which directs the environmentalist to evaluate the situation. If additional help is required, the environmentalist may secure the assistance of experts from top governmental agencies.

PUBLIC HEALTH NURSE

The public health nurse provides a link between the physician and the home. In her role as teacher-consultant she is in a position to identify infections acquired after discharge and may be the first to become aware of a staphylococcal epidemic in newborn infants in the community.

She serves as a significant agent in the control of disease since she is familiar with local laws, sources of communicable disease or infection, periods of incubation, and symptoms and duration. She also assists the board of health in setting up and maintaining proper isolation procedures.

The public health nurse is interested in the concept of total health care of the individual and his family and contributes nursing skills that results in improvement of conditions in the social and physical environment. She is associated with family health and well-baby clinics, in addition to working with the prevention and control of diseases such as tuberculosis and venereal diseases, as well as drug abuse.

SCHOOL NURSE

Hospitals and health agencies maintain a close contact with schools in the area, since they are directly affected when contagion develops in the public schools.

In the fall, the opening of the school term frequently occasions the spread of some type of communicable disease. The school nurse is an essential agent for the interpretation of evidence of contagion among schoolchildren and in taking steps to control it.

The school nurses play an important role in health education in the community. They are especially concerned with the sharp increase in the incidence of venereal diseases and drug abuse in the teen-age group, and they work closely with health agencies and facilities for prevention and control.

Recognizing that a healthy body and mind are the best insurance against infection or disease, emphasis is placed on both mental and physical health of the teacher and pupil.

INTERHOSPITAL INFECTION CONTROL COMMITTEE

Maximum individual and community health may be achieved in a community where hospitals have a close working relationship. This relationship may be supported in part through the development of an interhospital infection control committee.

The purpose of the committee is to ensure the highest quality in the control of infectious diseases through the coordination of infection prevention and control standards among hospitals in the community.

Organization

Much time and effort will be required to organize the committee and to keep it active, but the results justify these expenditures. The membership of the interhospital committee should be composed of a representative from each member hospital and from the local health office. These representatives should command the respect of the facility they represent, since the major function of the members is to serve as a liaison between the committee and the facility. The local health officer is an important member of the committee because he has a relationship with the patient's environment before and after hospitalization.

The scope of community needs will suggest the necessary number of committee members. At times, a limited number of active participants may function more efficiently as a voting group. However, an open-door policy should be observed, thereby making it possible for interested facilities to delegate additional ex-officio personnel.

Establishing guidelines

Early in the organizational plan, each representative should furnish the committee with information concerning the infection control program of his hospital. This should include all policies and procedures, the employee health service plan, educational programs relating to infection control, and the system of collecting and reporting surveillance data.

A subcommittee is then appointed to compile the collected data and to formulate a set of standards that may be used as general guidelines for the infection control manual of the individual hospital.

Areas where standardization may be beneficial

In many communities physicians serve more than one hospital. Standardization eliminates confusion.

1. Isolation cleaning techniques, isolation policies for various diseases, length of isolation time, method of terminating isolation, and the isolation categories of diseases
2. Method of determining whether an infection is nosocomial
3. Basic procedures for testing antibiotic sensitivities
4. Uniform reporting format or content, since all data may be compared by hospital representatives at each meeting
5. Basic procedures for employee health programs, including necessary immunizations and tests, and how often they are indicated
6. Infection control vocabulary
7. Cooperative infection control educational programs
8. Methods for reporting infections after the patient is discharged

Standardization is especially beneficial to physicians who service patients in several hospitals, since techniques of infection control will be similar.

Function

In no way does the interhospital infection control committee supplant the individual hospital's infection control committee. It serves as a valuable resource to offer practical help and stimulate interest.

The committee should hold monthly meetings to compare reports, discuss serious problems, share new ideas, and plan for the prevention of potential problems. A review of the standards and of the adequacy of current instruction and practices should be conducted periodically.

It is the aim of the committee to keep abreast of new techniques and endorse recommendations for better prevention and control of community- and hospital-associated infections.

CHAPTER SEVEN

Nursing care plans for the isolation patient

Systematic planning for care of the isolation patient is becoming more important as the nurse's role of responsibility in regard to the patient's total response to his illness becomes more complex. A written, personalized plan for each patient enables the nurse to share this responsibility with members of the patient care team by providing a basis for continuity of the teaching and care of the individual patient. The concept of planned care places the focus on the patient, sets priorities of care, upgrades nursing practices through systematic communication, and affords an opportunity for close observation of the patient as changes in his responses and attitudes occur.

Each patient is unique. Therefore, the nursing care plans offered here contain the basic factors peculiar to a specific disease or category of diseases that may be of value in determining needs and formulating individualized plans.

MENINGITIS, ESPECIALLY MENINGOCOCCAL
Respiratory category precautions

1. Observe and record
   a. Intracranial pressure
   b. Beginning of or increased nuchal rigidity
   c. Increased headache
   d. Elevated temperature
   e. Projectile vomiting
   f. Restlessness or irritability
   g. Lethargy or coma
   h. Increased photophobia
   i. Rash or hemorrhagic petechiae
2. Hygienic needs
   a. Frequent oral hygiene to prevent crusting or cracking of lips and mouth

     b. Hypothermia blanket to reduce febrile problems

     c. Air-water or foam mattress to prevent decubiti

3. Comfort measures

     a. Analgesics and antipyretics, as ordered by the physician

     b. Darkened room to ease headache and eye tension

     c. Quiet or soundproof room to prevent an increase of central nervous system irritation due to noise outside the room

     d. Ice cap on head to relieve surface tension

     e. Turn patient slowly and carefully to avoid excessive pain

4. Nutrition

     a. Accurate intake and output records (patient is generally receiving I.V. therapy)

     b. Patient kept well hydrated by giving frequent small amounts of fluid (only with physician's order)

     c. When solid food is permitted, an attractive tray with small-to-moderate amount of food

5. Safety measures

     a. Use of rectal thermometer, which is always necessary during acute phase to prevent patient from biting down on glass thermometer

     b. Padded side rails to prevent injury to patient during periods of irritability and confusion

     c. Padded tongue blades, taped to patient's bed to be used during seizure

6. Patient teaching

     a. Apprehension of family members relieved by explaining disease, its transmission, and methods of protecting themselves and others (initial explanations by the physician, after which the nursing staff answers questions as they are asked)

     b. Quiet and gentle approach to patient, with explanation of each procedure as it is being done

     c. Because patient may be very frightened by severe nightmares or strange body feelings, alleviation of fear through understanding and good verbal communication

     d. Instruction of visitors, family, and personnel in the proper respiratory precautions (both how and why)

TUBERCULOSIS
Respiratory category precautions

1. Observe and record

     a. Sputum—amount and color

     b. Nutritional status of patient

    c. Patient's acceptance or nonacceptance of the disease

    d. Family's fear and its relationship to patient

2. Hygienic needs
   a. Good oral and body hygiene
   b. Frequent change of sputum containers
   c. Proper use of the tissue technique in coughing or sneezing
   d. Sanitary environment
3. Comfort measures
   a. Bright, cheerful surroundings
   b. Opportunity for patient to rest and read as desired
   c. Outside walking and exercise permitted
   d. Abundant communications of family and friends
4. Nutrition
   a. Selective menu of nourishing foods
   b. For malnourished patient, use of between-meal supplements
   c. Dietary consultation to help patient select proper diet
5. Safety measures
   a. Mask worn by patient when others are present (or patient leaves the room) during period of communicability
   b. When mask is not worn, good tissue technique when patient coughs and sneezes
   c. Proper bagging and disposal of all sputum and containers
6. Patient, family, and visitor teaching
   a. Instruction of patient concerning nature of the disease, its transmission, and prevention of spread
   b. Proper tissue, mask, and handwashing techniques, with an understanding of both how and why; frequent checking on their use
   c. Instruction of family and visitors on correct use of masks and why; full instructions concerning handwashing procedures and why
   d. Patient and family allowed to ventilate feelings about the disease; use of this experience as a tool for teaching
   e. Instruction of family and patient on home care to be followed after discharge

TYPHOID FEVER
Enteric category precautions

1. Observe and record
   a. Signs of dehydration
   b. Rise in temperature
   c. Headache

    d. Generalized malaise or weakness

    e. Slow pulse

    f. Rose-colored rash on trunk or abdomen

    g. Chills

    h. Bloody diarrhea or constipation

    i. Gas and abdominal distension

    j. Signs of bowel perforation, pain, shock, etc.

2. Hygienic needs

    a. Rectal temperatures taken frequently

    b. Because patient often has either urinary retention or involuntary voidings, use of Foley catheter to prevent urinary spread of infection and to obtain an accurate record of urinary output

    c. Excellent oral hygiene to prevent mouth ulcers and cracking, bleeding lips

    d. Frequent position change to avoid skin irritation and breakdown

    e. Tepid baths to reduce fever

    f. Patient kept hydrated

    g. Accurate intake and output record

3. Comfort needs

    a. Frequent change of bed linen to avoid odor due to severe diaphoresis

    b. To prevent severe constipation, check the number, kind, and size of stools; enemas as needed (by physician's order)

    c. Use of sheepskin to prevent skin irritation from bed sheets

    d. Cool sponges, packs, or alcohol rubs to improve skin tone and stimulate patient's well-being

    e. Release of excess gas by insertion of rectal tube

    f. Chance for patient to ventilate his feelings

4. Nutrition

    a. Cold liquids, which are appealing during the fever stage of the disease

    b. Encouragement to eat

    c. Tasteful, attractive, bland, high-caloric diet

5. Safety measures during acute febrile stage

    a. Padded tongue blades taped to bed

    b. Side rails up since patient is drowsy and indifferent to surroundings

    c. Use of rectal thermometer

    d. Use of good handwashing technique to prevent disease spread

    e. Patient area kept free from flies

6. Teaching

    a. Visitors and relatives helped to understand how disease is spread; explanation of home precautions

   b. Explanation to the patient of each treatment as it is given and why

   c. Explanation to the patient why the body is reacting as it is and how it will respond to treatment and nutrition

   d. Instruction of visitors, relatives, and personnel on enteric technique, especially the importance of good handwashing

   e. Instruction of patient and family on home precautions

ENTERIC DISEASE (SALMONELLOSIS, SHIGELLOSIS, AND AMEBIC DYSENTERY)
Enteric category precautions

1. Observe and record
   a. Diarrhea: amount, kind, and color
   b. Abdominal cramps and distension
   c. Elevated temperature
   d. Headache or vomiting
   e. Prostration
   f. Chills, malaise, and generalized aching
   g. Slow pulse

2. Hygienic needs
   a. Adequate fluids to maintain proper acid-base and electrolyte balance
   b. Careful maintenance of correct intake and output
   c. Good oral hygiene during period of dehydration
   d. Good rectal hygiene to prevent skin excoriation

3. Comfort measures
   a. Keep patient and bed surroundings clean and dry
   b. Frequent use of ointment to rectal area to ease irritation due to frequent stools
   c. Insertion of rectal tube carefully to prevent flatus accumulation
   d. Provision of crushed ice or cool fluids to relieve oral dryness due to dehydration
   e. Provision of some room deodorizer to control room odors due to frequent defecation

4. Nutrition
   a. Frequent nourishing liquids to replace lost fluids
   b. Attractive and interesting tray when solids are provided
   c. All leftover food discarded in waste container; liquids discarded in the restroom commode

5. Safety
   a. Good handwashing technique after discarding of urine, feces, or food

    b. Use of ordinary safety precautions for patient care
6. Teaching
    a. Explanation to family of how disease is transmitted and erad-
       icated.
    b. Instruction of family, visitors, and patient in proper handwashing
       and proper method of handling and preparing food
    c. Instruction of patient in proper elimination technique
    d. Instruction of family and patients in home care after discharge

DRAINING WOUNDS WITH AIRBORNE PATHOGENS (COAGULASE-POSITIVE STAPHYLOCOCCUS AND BETA HEMOLYTIC STREPTOCOCCUS, GRADE A)
Wound and skin/respiratory category precautions

1. Observe and record
    a. Drainage: amount, color, odor, and location
    b. Condition of skin bordering drainage site
    c. Condition of suture area
    d. Elevated temperature
    e. Lethargy
    f. Pain, redness, or heat in incisional area
    g. Confusion and restlessness
2. Hygienic needs
    a. Frequent dressing changes, using excellent technique
       (1) Removal, cleansing, and replacement of dressing
       (2) Soiled dressing disposal
    b. Good skin care
    c. Hypothermia blanket if elevated temperature does not respond
       to medication
    d. Good handwashing technique, used frequently by patient, vis-
       itors, and personnel
3. Comfort measures
    a. Patient kept comfortable with analgesics and antipyretics as pre-
       scribed by physician
    b. Frequent linen changes if soiled by dressings
    c. Hot or cold packs kept at an even temperature
4. Nutrition
    a. Selective menu of patient's choice, high in protein, if permitted
       by physician
    b. Frequent nourishing liquids
    c. Provision of sufficient roughage in diet for natural body elimina-
       tion
5. Safety measures

    a. Prevention of cross contamination of wounds
      (1) Good handwashing technique
      (2) Proper dressing disposal technique
    b. Safety measures applicable to any postoperative patient
    c. Terminal room disinfection
6. Teaching
    a. Instruction of personnel who change dressings, regarding mask technique to prevent airborne spread of the disease
    b. Instruction of patient in the "hands off dressing" technique
    c. Review of handwashing procedure with personnel and visitors
    d. Review, with personnel, of all procedures of care that will prevent cross contamination

DRAINING WOUNDS WITH NONAIRBORNE PATHOGENS (PROTEUS, ESCHERICHIA COLI, PSEUDOMONAS)
Wound and skin category precautions

Use the same techniques as in draining wounds with airborne pathogens, with the following exceptions:
    a. No mask needed
    b. Semiprivate room or ward
    c. Mandatory excellent handwashing by nurse between patients
    d. Drainage limited to small or moderate amount
    e. Private room if drainage is copious, because of greater danger of contamination

GAS GANGRENE
Wound and skin category precautions

1. Observe and record
    a. Edema and gaseous infiltration at the wound site or the muscle surrounding the wound site
    b. Discoloration and tissue necrosis around or in the wound site
    c. Gaseous odor of hydrogen sulfide
    d. Frothy reddish brown wound discharge in early stages of the disease, followed by pus in the later stages
    e. Apathy, weakness, semicoma, or severe anemia
2. Hygienic needs
    a. Wound kept open, debrided, and well aerated
    b. Strict dressing technique both in changing dressings and in their disposal
    c. The patient and his surroundings kept clean at all times
    d. Good handwashing procedures frequently employed by patient and personnel

    e. Autoclaving of linen before being washed, or washed separately at high temperature

    f. Room vented to outside, with frequent air exchange

3. Comfort measures

    a. Quiet, clean, pleasing surroundings

    b. Patient kept informed about his treatments

    c. Use of analgesics as ordered by the physician to keep the patient free from pain

    d. Room deodorizers to reduce gas odors that emanate from the wound area

    e. Dressings kept clean and dry

4. Nutrition

    a. Well-balanced diet of the patient's selection

    b. Frequent nourishing liquids

    c. Frequent supplementary feedings to maintain proper body tissue buildup

5. Safety

    a. Incineration of all soiled dressings

    b. Autoclaving of all soiled linen before washing

    c. Incineration of all wastes from patient's room

    d. Mandatory excellent, frequent handwashing

    e. Gloves worn by personnel who change dressings

    f. Terminal disinfection of all articles that have become contaminated by the infective organism

6. Teaching

    a. Instruction of family and visitors as to proper precautions used while in the patient's room

       (1) Do not sit on the patient's bed

       (2) Do not touch the patient's linens or dressings

       (3) Wash hands before leaving the room

    b. Instruction of personnel on dressing removal and replacement

    c. Instruction of personnel on precautions to be used in waste removal

INFECTIOUS AND SERUM HEPATITIS
Enteric category precautions

1. Observe and record

    a. Jaundice (eyes and body)

    b. Urine (dark brown)

    c. Stools (clay-colored)

    d. Elevated temperature

    e. Abdominal discomfort

    f. Nausea, vomiting

    g. General malaise

    h. Unusual behavior after visiting hours (only in serum hepatitis)

    i. New needle marks on arms or legs

2. Hygienic needs

    a. Good oral and body hygiene

    b. Good patient handwashing after bathroom use and before eating

    c. Individual commode if patient is in a ward or semiprivate room

3. Comfort measures

    a. Quiet, pleasant surroundings

    b. Magazines or books to provide diversion during bed rest

    c. Medication to relieve nausea (as ordered by the physician)

4. Nutrition

    a. Nourishing low-fat liquids while patient is nauseated

    b. High-protein, low-fat meals in small quantity, which is increased as the nausea subsides and the patient develops an appetite (diet and approximate quantity will usually be indicated by physician and patient)

5. Safety

    a. Patient not permitted to eat in the hospital cafeteria

    b. Bathroom use limited to the one assigned to patient for his exclusive use

    c. Disinfection of bathroom or commode assigned to the patient before it can be used by someone else

    d. Terminal steam or gas sterilization of all bedpans and commodes

    e. Destruction of all thermometers used rectally by these patients

    f. Terminal disinfection of bathroom and the patient's room

6. Teaching

    a. Instruction of patient as to the nature of the disease and its residual effects

    b. Instruction of patient, personnel, and the patient's family

        (1) Importance of using sterile needles

        (2) Hazards of eating in substandard places

        (3) Methods of good handwashing before eating and after elimination

        (4) Danger of drinking from cup or glass that was previously used by another person

ENCEPHALITIS

1. Observe and record

    a. Signs of photophobia

   b. Extreme headaches
   c. Noise intolerance
   d. Agitation and restlessness
   e. Elevated temperature
2. Hygienic needs
   a. Good oral and body hygiene
   b. Frequent position change if patient is semicomatose to avoid skin breakdown
   c. Use of foam or water mattress
   d. Hypothermia blanket for elevated temperature
3. Comfort measures
   a. Use of analgesics and antipyretics as prescribed by the physician to alleviate headache and fever
   b. Patient's room kept cool, quiet, and dark
   c. Explanation of each treatment as given to allay patient's apprehension
   d. Avoidance of room shadows, if possible, since the patient may hallucinate
   e. Quiet speaking and working in the room; no sudden movements that may frighten the patient
4. Nutrition
   a. Intravenous or liquid diet; liquids pleasant in appearance and taste
   b. For convalescent patient, a light, nourishing diet, with changes as to consistency and content as the patient's needs dictate (physician should authorize any change in diet)
   c. Foods that encourage natural body elimination to avoid constipation
5. Safety
   a. Padded side rails to prevent the confused or convulsed patient from injury to himself
   b. Padded tongue blades taped to head of bed in case the patient has a convulsion
   c. Light restraints, with the physician's permission, or a member of the family in constant attendance, if the patient attempts to get out of bed
6. Teaching
   a. Instruction of personnel, family, and visitors as to the nature of the disease, and an explanation of the patient's response to the disease
   b. Review of each treatment with the patient before or during treatment

CHICKENPOX
Respiratory category precautions

1. Observe and record
   a. Elevated temperature
   b. Areas where the rash first appears and any new areas of invasion (rash usually appears first on the back)
   c. Stages of maturity of the rash, from maculopapular, to vesicular lesions, to scabs
   d. Headache and mild respiratory symptoms
   e. Complications
      (1) Pneumonia
      (2) Septic complication
      (3) Encephalitis (children)
2. Hygienic needs
   a. Good oral, body, and scalp cleanliness
   b. Gloves placed on the hands of young children to avoid scratching and infection
   c. Frequent linen changes to prevent reinfection of open pustules
3. Comfort measures
   a. Frequent warm baths to ease itching
   b. Lotion or ointment applied to rash areas to alleviate itching
   c. Oral or intramuscular medication as ordered by the physician to ease the discomfort of itching
   d. Cool liquids, taken orally, for elevated temperature
   e. Diversional therapy, especially for the young child
4. Nutrition
   a. Frequent nourishing liquids
   b. Diet as requested by the patient, tastefully prepared
   c. Foods that will ensure proper daily elimination
5. Safety measures
   a. Patient's room vented to the outside, and frequent air exchange (for prevention of cross contamination)
   b. Room kept under negative pressure to prevent the escape of air from the room when doors are opened or shut.
   c. Proper disinfection of all articles that are soiled by oral secretions of patient
   d. Terminal disinfection of the room and furniture

Glossary

acquired immunity Process by which the body builds up resistance to certain pathogens.

active immunity Process by which the body manufactures its own antibodies.

aerobe Any organism that lives only in the presence of free oxygen.

alert category Classification of a group of infectious diseases; designed to provide temporary safe care for patients with probable or undiagnosed disease or infection until diagnosis is confirmed.

amoeba Simple form of animal life.

anaerobe Any microorganism capable of living without free air or oxygen.

antibody Specific chemical substance formed by the cells of the organism; has the capacity to react to the invasion by antigens.

antidote Substance that prevents poison from acting on cells when it is introduced into the body.

antigen Substance that causes the body's defense mechanism when introduced into the body to produce antibodies.

antiseptic Chemical agent that inhibits microbial growth; the term is often used for agents that act on organisms associated with the body.

antitoxin Substance produced in the body to overcome the poison of disease.

arthropod Member of the group of vectors having paired, jointed legs and capable of transmitting disease to man.

asepsis Absence of pathogenic organisms from a given area.

attenuated Weakened or rendered inactive.

autoclave Equipment used for sterilizing medical supplies by means of steam under pressure.

bacillus Rod-shaped bacterium.

bacteria Microorganisms; microscopic forms of life that spread universally in nature.

bactericidal Pertaining to a chemical agent that kills bacteria.

bacteriostatic Pertaining to a chemical agent that prevents microbes from multiplying; term is frequently used in referring to the action of certain antibiotics.

biologic transmission Transmission from host to host by an animal or insect in which the organism undergoes a cycle of development in the vector's body before it is transmitted.

botulism Food poisoning by the bacillus.

carrier Person without symptoms of a communicable disease who harbors and disseminates an infective organism.

coccus (cocci) Spherical-shaped bacterium.

communicable Able to be spread from one to another.

concurrent disinfection Destruction of pathogenic organisms as soon as possible after they have been discharged from the infected person.

contagious disease Disease that can be transmitted by contact or inhalation.

contamination Presence of organisms that might cause infectious conditions.

control In the hospital setting, prevention of the spread of an already existing infection or disease.

cross infection A second communicable disease superimposed on the first.

culture Growth of microbes on or in nutrient substances.

diphtheroids Nonpathogenic organisms resembling the diphtheria bacillus.

disinfectant Chemical that destroys pathogenic microorganisms.

dysentery Intestinal infection resulting in persistent diarrhea.

endemic Pertaining to disease that is constantly present in a region but does not spread to other regions.

endogenous Developing from within the body.

enteric Pertaining to diseases caused by pathogenic feces and urine.

epidemic Pertaining to a disease that affects many people in an area and spreads rapidly.

epidemiology (*epi,* "upon"; *demi,* "people"; *logy,* "study") Science that deals with incidence, distribution, and control of disease in a population.

exanthem Skin rash occurring in some communicable diseases.

exogenous Pertaining to infection resulting from contamination by a source outside the body.

focal infection Infection confined to a restricted area.

fomites Contaminated objects by which disease-producing organisms are spread.

fungi Microscopic plant life of mold forms.

fungicide Chemical agent that destroys fungi.

germicide Chemical agent that destroys microorganisms.

host Human, animal, or inanimate object having a pathogen present on or within the body.

immunity Body's resistance to disease; may be active, passive, natural, or acquired.

incubation period Time between infection and the appearance of signs or symptoms of the disease.

infection Establishment of a pathogen in its host after invasion; contagious or infectious disease.

isolation Separation of a patient and his immediate surroundings from all other people to prevent the spread of disease organisms.

lesion Wound or local degeneration.

localized infection Infection confined to a particular body area.

mechanical transmission The infected organism adheres to a vector's body and is carried from place to place.

microbe Smallest living being.

microbiology Study of organisms too small to be seen without a microscope.

microorganism Minute plant or animal.

microscope Optical instrument for making enlarged images of minute objects.

morbidity Sick rate.

morphology Structure or form of an organism.

nosocomial infection Hospital-associated infection.

pathogen Disease-producing organism.

pathogenic Pertaining to disease or infection producers.

petri dish Flat dish used for culturing in the laboratory.

prevention Protection of the uninfected patient from disease for the purpose of forestalling any increase in preexisting infection of a noncommunicable disease.

protect To shield from injury or destruction.

purulent Containing pus.

pyogenic bacteria Pus-forming bacteria.

quarantine Limitation of movement of persons or animals who have been exposed to communicable disease.

resistance Ability to resist disease.

reverse category Classification of highly susceptible patients having no infectious disease but needing protection from pathogens of others.

Schick test Skin test to detect susceptibility to diphtheria.

sepsis Bacteriologic process of decay.

septicemia Diseased condition due to the presence of pathogenic bacteria in the bloodstream.

specimen Sample of material taken from the body and examined in a laboratory to identify a disease or its cause.

sterile Free from living organisms.

strict category Classification of a group of infectious diseases; designed to protect personnel and patients from highly communicable airborne diseases.

surveillance Close supervision of a person, disease, or condition; necessary for control of infection.

symptoms Manifestations of a disease felt by the patient.

terminal cleaning Thorough cleaning of a room and its contents after discharge of an isolation patient.

terminal disinfection Killing of all organisms that might still be found on articles after isolation has been discontinued.

trimester A period of three months; in obstetrics, the first, second, or third three-month period of pregnancy.

tuberculin test Skin test to determine tubercular infection.

vaccination Protective inoculation against a disease.

vector A carrier, especially the animal host (usually an arthropod) that carries an infective agent from one person to another.

wound and skin category Classification of a group of infectious diseases; designed to protect personnel and patients where pathogens exist in wounds or skin infections.

Index

A

Active immunity, 16
Admission
  of isolation patient to recovery room, 80
  of isolation patient to x-ray department, 71
  of patient to isolation, 45-48
    door card, 47
    order for, 45
    pediatric, 45
    room, preparation for, 45
  as source of data collection, 115
Airborne diseases; *see* Nursing care plans; Respiratory category of diseases
Alert category of isolation, 88-90
Amebic dysentery; *see also* Enteric category of isolation
  nursing care plans for, 142
American Hospital Association, 132
Antibiotics, indiscriminate use of, 10
Antigen-antibodies, 16; *see also* Immunity

B

Bacteria, 1-4
  morphology, 3-4
    cocci, 3
    bacilli, 4
    spiral, 4
  optimum conditions for growth, 1
    cycle, 1
    phases, 2
    oxygen requirements, 3
    pH, 3
    temperature, 3
  reproduction of, 4
  sporulation of, 4
  staining of, 4
    gram-negative, 4
    gram-positive, 4

Blood pressure
  isolation policy and procedure for taking of, 57
  sphygmomanometer
    enteric precautions for, 91
    respiratory precautions for, 94
    strict precautions for, 95
Body
  care of, after death, 77-78
  natural defenses against pathogens, 14-16
    chemical protection, 15
    conjunctiva, 14
    gastrointestinal tract, 15
    genitourinary system, 15
    immunity, 16
    inflammation, 15
    lungs, 15
  resistance lowered, 14
  site of normal flora, 5 (table)
Books in strict isolation category, 96
Brochure for dissemination of information on isolation procedures, 127
Buzz sessions, 106; *see also* Educational program

C

Capsules of pathogens, 10
Card; *see* specific categories of isolation for door card legends
  nosocomial case, 118-119
Cardiac resuscitation; *see* Code-arrest cart
Carriers of infections, 12
  convalescent, 12
Cart
  for use when cleaning isolation areas, 74
  code-arrest, in isolation, 72
  isolation supply, 46
Categories of isolation, 82-100
  alert, 88-90

Categories of isolation—cont'd
  enteric, 90-92
  respiratory, 92-94
  reverse, 99-100
  strict, 94-97
    smallpox, 96
  wound and skin, 97-99
Catheter
  intravenous therapy, 34
  urinary care, 37
CDC; *see* Center for Disease Control
Center for Disease Control
  classifications of infections by, 17-18
  educational programs offered by, 110
  in relation to health services, 132
  training bulletin of, 110; *see also* Educational program
Central service
  equipment in; *see* Equipment
  gas sterilization, 67-68
  steam sterilization, 67
  thermometers cleaned by, 68
Certification of continuing education programs, 110
Chart, patient's
  indications of infection for data purposes, 113
  in isolation, policies and procedures for, 48
  strict category, 95
Checklist for program planners, 103; *see also* Educational program
Chickenpox, nursing care plans for, 148
Classification of infections, 17-18
  gastrointestinal, 17
  others, 17
  respiratory, 17
  urinary tract, 17
  wound and skin, 17
Cleaning
  alert precautions, 90
  cultures, 77
  enteric precautions, 92
  emergency room, after isolation patient removed, 80
  environmental services department, 39
  final inspection, 76
  general cleaning, 39-40
  initial cleaning, 74-76
  Isolettes, 44
  multiple occupancy units with probable contamination, 77
  operating room between cases, 39-40
  respiratory precautions in, 94
  reverse precautions in, 100
  strict precautions in, 96

Cleaning—cont'd
  terminal, 74-77
  wound and skin precautions in, 99
  x-ray department, 41
Clinic in educational programs, 107
Clothing and personal effects in strict category of isolation, 96
Code-arrest cart, 72
  nursing service personnel responsible for, 73
  respiratory therapist responsible for, 73
Coding of data; *see* Data
Comfort measures; *see* nursing care plans for specific diseases
Committee
  infection control, 19-24
  interhospital, 135-137
Community-associated infections, 16-17
Conference, 106; *see also* Emotional needs of patients
Control; *see also* Categories of isolation
  definition of, x
  policies and procedures for, 45-82
Cultures
  prevention policies and procedures, 36-37
  routine in operating and delivery rooms, 39
  of terminally cleaned isolation room, 77
  wound and skin category of isolation, 99

D

Data, 111-123; *see also* Nurse epidemiologist, functions
  assimilation of, 118
    by monthly report, 118
    by nosocomial case card, 118
  coding of, 115
  collection of, 112-118
    daily, 115-118
      in admitting department, 115
      on daily discharge sheet, 116
      on incident report of infection, 116, 117
      in laboratory, 116
      from physician's office, 118
      in ward rounds, 116
      in x-ray department, 116
    indications of infection on patient's chart or departmental reports, 113, 114
  responsibility for, 112

Data—cont'd
  collection of—cont'd
    sources of, 115
    tools for, 115
  on handling a nursery outbreak, 121
  interpretation of, 120
  on investigation of hospital-associated
    epidemics, 121
  problem solving by use of, 120
  purpose for reporting of, 112
    general, 112
    specific, 112
Death, care of body after, 77, 78
Deep breathing in prevention of infec-
    tions, 39
Defenses; see Body
Demonstration assignment in educational
    programs, 106
Dietary service
  dishes and food, category precautions
    alert, 89
    enteric, 91
    respiratory, 94
    strict, 96
    wound and skin, 99
  feeding infants, 42-43
  to isolation patients, 57-58
Direct transfer of infections, 13
Discharge of patient
  from isolation to home, 78
  remaining in same room after isola-
    tion, 79
  transfer to another room after, 78
Discharge sheet as daily source of data
    collection, 116
Discussion; see also Educational program
  panel, 105
  sectional, 106
Diseases
  categories of, 88-100; see also Cate-
    gories of isolation
  general list, category and duration of,
    83-88
  nursing care plans for, 138-148
  reportable to public health department,
    122-123
Dishes; see Dietary service
Documents, signing of, 62-63
Door card
  in admission policy, 47
  legends in isolation categories
    alert, 88
    enteric, 90
    respiratory, 92
    reverse, 100

Door card—cont'd
  legends in isolation categories—cont'd
    strict, 94
    wound and skin, 98
Double bagging
  of dressings, 58
  of equipment, 66
    for gas sterilization, 67
    for steam sterilization, 67
    respiratory therapy, used by, 68
  of food and disposable utensils, 58
  of linen, 59-61
Drainage system, closed, 37
Dressings
  control policies and procedures for, 58
    double bagging of, 58
  precautions for, in isolation categories
    alert, 89
    enteric, 91
    respiratory, 94
    strict, 96
    wound and skin, 99
  prevention policies and procedures for,
    36
Draining wounds; see Wound
Droplet, infection by, 13
Drugs; see Medications
Duodenum, normal flora of, 8

E

Educational program, 101-111
  aids to leaders of, 104
  Center for Disease Control, programs
    offered, 110
  certification of continuing education,
    110
  checklist for planners of, 103
  evaluation of, 111
  instructors for, 101
  introduction of speakers, 103
  methods for presenting of, 104-107
    buzz session, 106
    clinic, 107
    conference, 106
    demonstration assignments, 106
    forum, 106
    lecturing, 105
    panel, 105
    role play, 105
    sectional discussion, 106
    seminar, 106
    skits, 105
    symposium, 105
    workshop, 107
  participants for, 102
  planning of, 102

Educational program—cont'd
  posters and memorandums in, 110
  types of, 107-110
    general program, 108
    hospital orientation, 107
    on-the-spot teaching, 110
    unit and departmental teaching, 109
Electrocardiogram equipment in isolation, 69
Emergency room
  care of patients with communicable disease, 80
  cleaning, after isolation patient, 80
  isolation patient admitted to hospital from, 80
Emotional needs
  of family, 126, 127
  met through brochures of information, 127
  of patients, 124-127
    pediatric, 125
    teen-ager, 126
Encephalitis nursing care plans, 146, 147
Endemic, 10-11
Endogenous organisms, 12
Endotoxins, 19
Enteric category of isolation, 90-92
Enteric disease nursing care plans, 140, 142, 145, 146
Environmentalist in public health service, 133, 134
Environmental service department; see Housekeeping
Epidemic
  definition of, 10, 11
  hospital-associated, 121
  nursery outbreak, 121
Epidemiologist
  hospital, 21
  nurse, 22, 24; see also Nurse
Epidemiology
  endemic disease and, 10, 11
  endogenous organisms and, 12
  epidemic and, 10, 11
  exogenous organisms and, 12
  of infection, 10, 11
  pandemic and, 10
  sequences of factors in, 11
Equipment
  for central service, 66-73
  electrocardiogram, 69
  ice machines and scoops, 33-34
  respiratory, 68
  nonpiped-in oxygen, 68
  piped-in oxygen, 69
  special instruments and trays, 91

Equipment—cont'd
  for terminal cleaning of isolation room, 74
  thermometers, 33, 68
  traction, 70
  x-ray, 72
Evaluation of programs, 111
Excreta, precautions for in isolation categories
  alert, 89
  enteric, 91
  respiratory, 94
Exogenous organisms, 12
Exotoxins, 9
Eyedrops, one-unit dosage, 39

F

Family, emotional needs of, 126, 127
Flora, normal, 5-9
Fomites, 13
Food; see also Dietary service
  feeding infants, 42
Forum in educational programs, 106

G

Gas gangrene, nursing care plans for, 144
Gastrointestinal tract
  body's natural defenses of, 15
  classifications of infections of, 17
  normal flora of, 9
Gathering of data; see Data, collection of
Genitourinary tract
  body's natural defenses of, 15
  normal flora, 9
Gloves
  control policies and procedures, 52-55
    nonsterile, 52
    sterile, 52
  precautions for in isolation categories
    alert, 89
    enteric, 91
    reverse, 99
    strict, 95
    wound and skin, 99
Gowns
  control policies and procedures, 49-52
    in pediatrics, 49
  precautions for, 89, 91, 93, 95, 99, 100
Gram, Hans Christian; see Staining of bacteria
Growth cycle of bacteria, 1, 2

H

Health services
  American Hospital Association, 132
  Center for Disease Control, 132
  interhospital infection control commit-
      tee, 135-137
    function, 136
    guidelines, 136
    organization, 135
    standardization areas, 136
  nurse in
    personnel health services, 27
    public, 134
    school, 135
  personnel, 26
  public health service, 133
    environmentalist, 133
Handwashing policy and procedure, 29-
    32, 49
Hepatitis, infectious and serum, 145-146,
    90-92
High-risk areas and isolation
  emergency room, 79-80
  intensive care unit, 79
  nursery, 82
  recovery room, 80
  surgery, 81
Hospital-acquired infections, 131
Hospital-associated infections, 16, 17
Host
  as infectious agent, 11
  in mode of transmission, 14
Housekeeping
  general cleaning, 39
  terminal cleaning of isolation room,
      74-77
Hyaluronidase, 10
Hygienic needs; *see* nursing care plans
    for specific diseases
Hyperalimentation, 34

I

Ice scoops and machines, 33, 34
Immunity
  active, 16
  antigen-antibodies, 16
  body's natural defenses, 16
  charitable, 129
  government, 129
  immunization, 16
  passive, 16
  vaccination, 16
Immunization, 16
  personnel health services program, 26
Immunosuppressive drugs, 14
Inanimate sources of infection, 12

Incident report of infection, 116
Indications of infections on patient's
    chart, 113, 114
Indirect contact of infections, 13
Infection control committee
  functions of, 21, 22
  membership of, 21-23
  recommendations for, 19-21
Infections
  carriers of, 12
  classification of, 17, 18
  community-associated, 16, 17
  epidemiology of, 10-12
  hospital-acquired, 131
  hospital-associated, 16, 17
  indications of, 113, 114
  interrupting sequence of, 16
  legal aspects of, 128-131
  nosocomial, 16, 17
  signs of in nursery, 42
  sources, 12, 13
  transfer of, 13
Infectious hepatitis, 145-146
Inflammation, 15
Information, coding, 115; *see also* Bro-
    chure
Instructors for educational programs, 101
Intensive care, 43, 79
Interhospital committee, 135-137
Interpretation of data, 120
Intramuscular injections, 43, 62
Intravenous therapy
  catheter, 34
  hyperalimentation, 34
  infusion of isolation patient, 62
  prevention policies, procedures, 34, 35
Investigation of hospital-associated epi-
    demic, 121
Isolette cleaning, 44

K

Kinases, 10

L

Laboratory; *see* Data, daily collection of;
    Specimens
Laundry; *see also* Linen
  handling clean linen in, 39
  handling contaminated linen in, 59-61
    double bagging, 59
Lecturing in educational programs, 105
Legal aspects of infection, 128-131
  charitable immunity and, 129
  circumstances in, 130, 131
  government immunity and, 129
  hospital-acquired infections and, 131

Legal aspects of infection—cont'd
  res ipsa loquitor and, 129
  respondeat superior and, 129
  torts and, 128
Linen; *see also* Laundry
  clean, 39
  double bagging of, 59-61
  precautions for; *see* Categories of isolation
  soiled, 38
  on stretcher or wheelchair, 73, 74
Lungs
  body's natural defenses in, 15
  normal flora in, 7

M

Mail, in isolation, 63, 96
Manual, 28, 29; *see also* Policies and procedures of control
Masks
  control policies and procedures, 49, 50
  precautions for; *see* Categories of isolation
  used in transportation of isolation patient, 73
Medications
  injections and infusions, 34, 43, 61-62
  oral, for isolation patient, 61
Meeting emotional needs of isolation patients, 124-127
Memorandums in educational programs, 110
Meningitis, nursing care plans for, 138
Methods
  of data collection, 113
  for presenting programs, 104-107
Microbiology, definition of, 1
Microorganisms and infection, 1-18
Mode of transmission, 13-14
  direct transfer as, 13
  droplets as, 13
  fomites as, 13
  host as, 13
  indirect contact as, 13
  portals of entry and exit as, 14
  vectors as, 13, 14
  vehicles as, 13
Money, handling of, in isolation, 62
Morphology of bacteria, 3
Mouth, normal flora of, 7

N

Nasopharynx, normal flora of, 7
Needles and syringes, precautions in categories of isolation
  alert, 89

Needles and syringes, precautions in categories of isolation—cont'd
  enteric, 91
  strict, 95
Normal flora, 5-9
  by body sites, 5-9
    duodenum, 8
    genitourinary tract, 9
    mouth, 7
    nasopharynx, 7
    other areas, 9
    skin, 9
    stomach, 7
    throat, 7
    trachea, bronchi, lungs, accessory nasal and mastoid sinuses, 7
  by resident microbes, 5 (table)
Nosocomial infections, 16, 17
  case card for, 118, 119
Nurse
  epidemiologist, 22, 23
    functions, 24
    member of infection control committee, 22
    qualifications of, 23
    role of, 22
  infection control, 22-23
  personnel health service, 27
  public health, 134
  role in surveillance program, 25
  school, 135
Nursery
  feeding in, 42, 43
  handling outbreaks in, 121
  intramuscular injections, 43
  isolation, 82
  Isolette cleaning, 44
  personnel in, 32, 41
  physician's examination in, 43
  policies and procedures of prevention in, 41-45
  signs of infection in, 42
Nursing care plans, 138-148
  chickenpox, 148
  draining wounds with airborne pathogens, 143
  draining wounds with nonairborne pathogens, 144
  encephalitis, 146-147
  enteric diseases, 142
  gas gangrene, 144-145
  hepatitis, infectious and serum, 145, 146
  meningitis, 138, 139
  tuberculosis, 139, 140
  typhoid fever, 140-141

Nutrition; *see* Dietary service; Nursing care plans for specific diseases

O

On-the-spot teaching, 110
Operating room; *see also* Surgery
  culture routine, 39
  cleaning between cases, 41
Oral suction, 35-36
Orientation, educational program, 107
Oxygen
  influence on microorganisms' growth, 3
  equipment in isolation, 68, 69

P

Pandemic, 10
Panel discussion, 105
Participants in educational programs, 102
Passive immunity, 16
Pathogens, 9-10
  airborne, 143; *see also* Respiratory category of diseases
  endotoxins, 9
  exotoxins, 9
  staphylococcus, 3, 8, 10
  toxins, 9
Patient
  admission to isolation, 45-48
  chart, 48
  discharge from isolation, 78, 79
  in emergency room, 80
  meeting emotional needs of, 124-127
  nursing care plans for, 138-148
  in recovery room, 80
  transportation, 73
  in x-ray department, 71
Pediatric, 45, 49, 125
Personnel
  cleaning of isolation rooms by, 74
  code-arrest cart, 73
  control policies and procedures, 56, 71, 81
  health service program, 26-28
    follow-up, 26
    immunizations in, 26
    nurse in, 27
    preemployment examinations, 26
    records in, 28
  infection prevention policies and procedures, 32, 33, 41
pH, influence on bacterial growth, 3
Phases of bacterial growth cycle, 2
Planning of programs, 102
Physician
  examination of infants by, 43

Physician—cont'd
  office as source in data collection, 118
  role in surveillance program, 25
Policies and procedures of control, 45-82
  admission of patient, 45-48
    preparation of room, 45-46
  blood pressure, taking of, 57
  body, care of, after death, 77
  chart, patient's, 48
  dietary service, 57-58
  discharge of isolation patient, 78, 79
  documents, signing of, 63
  dressings, 58
  equipment, 66-73
    code-arrest cart, 72
    electrocardiogram, 69
    oxygen, 68
    respiratory therapy, 68
    sterilization of
      gas, 67
      steam, 67
    thermometers, 68
    traction, 70
    x-ray, 71-72
  gloves, 52
  gowns, 49-52
  handwashing, 49
  laboratory, 63, 64
  linen, 59-61
    contaminated, handling, in laundry, 61
    double bagging, 59
  mail, 62
  masks, 49, 73
  medication, 61-62
    injections, 62
    intravenous infusion, 62
    oral, 61
  money, handling of, 62
  nursery isolation, 82
  pediatrics, 49
  personnel, 56
  pulse, taking of, 56
  respiration, taking of, 56
  specimens, collection of, 63-64
    blood, 65-66
    stool, 65
    urine
      single, 64
      24-hour, 64
  surgery, 81
  temperature, taking of, 56
  transportation, 73
  visitors, 55, 56
  waste, 59
  x-ray room, 71

Policies and procedures of prevention, 28-45
  catheter, 34
  cleaning, 39-40
    environmental services department, 39
    Isolette, 44
  cultures, 36-37
  definition of, 28
  dressings, 36
  equipment and supplies, 33
  handwashing, 29-32
    surgical scrub, 32
  ice scoops and machines, 33, 34
  intramuscular injections, 43
  intravenous therapy, 34
  hyperalimentation, 34
  linen, 38, 39
  nursery, 41-45, 121-122
  oral suction, 35, 36
  personnel, 32, 33
  tracheostomy care in nursery, 44
  urinary system, 37
    clean voided urine specimens, 38
  ventilation, 33
  visitors, 33
Portals of entry and exit, 14
Posters used in teaching methods, 110
Prevention; see also Policies and procedures of prevention
  deep breathing in, 39
  definition of, x
Problem solving through data, 120
Procedures; see also Policies and procedures of prevention
  definition of, 28
  manual of, 28, 29
  writing of, 28
Program; see Surveillance; Educational program
Public health service, 133-137
  environmentalist, 133
  hospital sanitarian, 133
  nurse, 134
Pulse, taking of, 56

R

Records; see nursing care plans for specific diseases; Personnel health service program
Recovery room, 80
Removal of patient from isolation, 78, 79
Reportable diseases, 122, 123
Reporting system; see Data
Reports, 113, 114, 116
Reproduction process of bacteria, 4

Resident microbes, 5 (table)
Resistance of body to pathogens, 14
Respiratory
  category of diseases, 92-94
  classification of infections, 17
  equipment, 68, 69
  isolation patient in recovery room, 80
  isolation patient in transportation, 73
Resuscitation, cardiac; see Code-arrest cart
Reverse category of isolation, 99-100
Role play, 105
Room, 45, 71, 80; see also Categories of isolation for specific door card legends

S

Safety measures; see Nursing care plans for specific diseases; policies and procedures under specific subject
Salmonellosis; see also Enteric category of isolation
  nursing care plans for, 142
Sanitarian, hospital, 133
School nurse, 135
Seminar, 106
Serum hepatitis, 145-146; see also Enteric category of isolation
Shigellosis, nursing care plan for, 142
Site, body; see Normal flora
Skits, 105
Skin
  normal flora of, 9
  unbroken skin in body's natural defenses, 14
  and wound category of isolation; see Wound
Sources of infection, 5, 12, 13, 115
Speakers, introduction of, 103
Specific purpose for reporting, 112
Specimens
  clean voided urine, 37-38
  collection of, 63, 64, 65, 66
  precautions for, in categories of isolation; see Categories of isolation
Sphygmomanometer; see Blood pressure
Sporulation of bacteria, 4
Staining of bacteria, 4
Standardization
  by American Hospital Association, 19
  by interhospital infection control committee, 136
  by Joint Commission on Accreditation of Hospitals, 19
Staphylococcus, 3, 8, 10

Sterilization, 9, 67
Stomach, normal flora, 7
Strict category of isolation, 94-97
Suction, oral, 36
Surgery; *see also* Operating room
  portable x-ray equipment in, 72
  scrubs, 32
  septic cases in, 81
Surveillance program, development of,
    25-124
  by categories of isolation, 82-99
  by data collection, assimilation and in-
      terpretation, 111-120
  by education, 101-111
  by personnel health service, 26-28
  by policies and procedures, 28-81
  role of nurse in, 25
  role of physician in, 25
Symposium, 105

T

Tabulating data, 118
Teaching
  education aids, 104
  patient; *see* nursing care plans for spe-
      cific diseases
Teen-ager, meeting emotional needs of,
    126
Temperature; *see also* Thermometers
  influence on bacterial growth, 2
  taking of, 56
Terminal disinfection; *see* Cleaning
Thermometers; *see also* Temperature
  in central service, 68
  precautions in categories, 89, 91, 94,
    95
Throat, normal flora of, 7
Tissues; *see* precautions for under spe-
    cific categories of isolation
Tools for collecting data, 115
Toxins, 9
Trachea, normal flora of, 7
Tracheostomy care in nursery, 44
Traction, 70

Transfer of patient, 78
Transmission; *see* Mode of transmission
Transportation, 73, 90, 91, 94, 97, 99,
    100
Tuberculosis, nursing care plans for, 139
Typhoid fever, nursing care plans for,
    140

U

Unit and departmental teaching, 109
Urinary closed drainage system, 37
Urinary classification of infection, 17

V

Vaccination, 16
Vectors of infection, 13, 14
Vehicles of infection, 13
Ventilation, 33
Visitors
  control policies and procedures, 55, 56
  prevention policies and procedures, 33
  precautions; *see* specific categories of
      isolation

W

Ward rounds as source of data collection,
    116
Waste, 58; *see also* Excreta, precautions
    for, in isolation categories
  of baskets, 59
  of body, 59
Workshops for training programs, 107
Wound
  classification of infections, 17
  nursing care plans for, 143, 144
  and skin category of isolation, 97-99

X

X-ray department
  admission of patient to, 71
  cleaning of, 41
  equipment in, 71, 72
  as source of data collection, 116